# Keeping Control

# KEEPING CONTROL

## Understanding and Overcoming Fecal Incontinence

*Marvin M. Schuster, M.D., and*
*Jacqueline Wehmueller*

*The Johns Hopkins University Press*
*Baltimore and London*

© 1994 The Johns Hopkins University Press
All rights reserved
Printed in the United States of America on acid-free paper
03 02 01 00 99 98 97 96 95 94      5 4 3 2 1

The Johns Hopkins University Press
2715 North Charles Street, Baltimore, Maryland 21218-4319
The Johns Hopkins Press Ltd., London

ISBN 0-8018-4915-2      ISBN 0-8018-4916-0 (pbk)

Library of Congress Cataloging in Publication Data will be found
at the end of this book.
A catalog record for this book is available from the British Library.

Illustrations by Jacqueline Schaffer

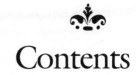

# Contents

# Prologue

*We wrote this book to provide information, so that you might gain a better understanding of fecal incontinence—what causes it and what can be done about it. But we also wrote this book to provide hope, because hope keeps people going. It's what gives them the attitude they need to change their situation.*

*If you have hope, you will seek help, and you will accept help that's offered to you. If you have hope, you won't give up. And, as you'll learn in this book, there's much to be hopeful about when it comes to the treatment of fecal incontinence.*

*This prologue is dedicated to Diane, a young woman who recently overcame a lifelong problem with fecal incontinence. We think that her story will inspire you—that it will give you hope.*

Diane was born with spina bifida, a condition in which the spinal cord is not completely closed over with tissue and skin. Early surgery protected Diane from infection and created a better cosmetic appearance, but the surgery couldn't undo all the other damage involved with her condition. It couldn't provide Diane's nerves with the connections they needed to communicate with one another, or with her muscles. As a result, Diane had some physical problems. For one thing, her nerves didn't give her muscles enough warning when she needed to go to the bathroom. Diane was not able to control when or where she urinated or defecated.

Despite her physical problems, Diane was a bright and happy child. She uncomplainingly wore diapers to catch urine long past the age when most children are toilet trained, and she cooperated in carrying out a routine designed to control her bowel movements. To minimize the chance that Diane would have a bowel movement in public, her parents gave Diane regularly scheduled enemas, and she would usually defecate at home. But Diane still had accidents, and as she got older the accidents became more embarrassing and more difficult to manage.

By the time she entered middle school, Diane had physically outgrown diapers, and whenever she urinated she had to change all her clothes. These accidents consumed so much of her time and emotional energy that the decision was made to remove Diane's urinary bladder and construct an artificial bladder for her. After this surgery, a bag attached to an opening on her abdomen collected urine, and Diane no longer wet herself.

Fecal incontinence continued to be a problem, however. Despite her enema regimen, at least once a week she would accidentally deposit stool into her underwear. Physical activity such as running made it more likely that she would have an accident, so in high school she couldn't take part in all the activities she wanted to.

In her twenty-third year, Diane had a job she enjoyed. She never dated, however, because she was afraid that she would have an accident while she was on a date and that the other person wouldn't understand. By this time she was finding it more and more difficult to cope with the enema regimen. She worried a lot about accidents, too, and if she had even a touch of diarrhea she would stay home from work, because with diarrhea she had little chance of controlling her bowels.

Diane began to consider having surgery to create an artificial opening for the collection of stool (a colostomy), just as she had earlier had surgery to create an opening for the collection of urine. While she was looking into what was involved with having this surgery, however, Diane talked to a doctor who suggested that she try a relatively new treatment for fecal incontinence, called *biofeedback training*. In biofeedback training, people learn to become aware of the body's signals, and to respond appropriately to them, by watching a visual representation of the energy output of their muscles which is displayed on an electronic recorder.

Diane's life changed dramatically when she decided to try this treatment. For the first time in her life, she learned to sense when there was stool in her rectum, and then she learned how to voluntarily contract her sphincters when she felt that sensation. After only one biofeedback session, Diane gained nearly total control of her bowels, and after the second session she had total control. Diane's success story is shared by many people who have turned to biofeedback training for help in overcoming fecal incontinence. The improvement is nearly always immediate, and the results are usually permanent.

It has now been three years since Diane had her biofeedback training, and she has not had a single accident. Her life has changed in many ways. For one thing, she can devote her full attention to her work and has recently moved into a new, more challenging position. Since physical activity no longer gives her problems, she's taken up many sports, like volleyball, that she'd never been able to do before. She's happily dating someone she met in a volleyball tournament. And she spends a lot of time thinking about the future.

# CHAPTER ONE

# What It Means to Be Incontinent

Most people take bowel control for granted. They go to work, run an errand, participate in sports, or enjoy an evening's entertainment—without ever once worrying about soiling their underwear with stool or, worse, having an accident so serious that people around them will notice the odor or the stain. But the fear of just such an accident causes some people to avoid working outside the home, to give up their weekly night out with friends, or even to miss an event as important as their child's wedding.

People with fecal incontinence lose liquid or solid stool or gas involuntarily from the anus at inappropriate times. Some people involuntarily pass small amounts of loose stool or mucus while passing gas, and some people evacuate their bowels into their clothing without any warning that they needed to have a bowel movement. Many people, especially older people, have no control over flatulence; this can be very embarrassing, too. If you are a person who has any of these problems, or if you are close to such a person, this book is for you.

However severe your problem is, and however long you've had it, this book may give you the hope you need to seek a cure.

Whether your problem is so slight that you have been managing it on your own or whether it is more severe, whether you have had this problem for a long time or whether it is new for you, fecal incontinence is probably affecting your life in many ways. You may stay home all the time, for example, because you need to stay close to a toilet. Or you may avoid developing close friendships or intimate relationships with other people because you're afraid they'll find out about your problem and disapprove of you if they do.

Just as devastating as social isolation is the way incontinence affects a person's self-esteem and well-being. Control of bowel and bladder function is the first form of self-control that we develop as young children. Because the control of bodily functions is such a basic ability, it is easy to understand why loss of sphincter control is often associated in a person's mind with loss of self-control. If you can't regulate this aspect of your environment (*yourself*), you may begin to feel that you can't regulate *any part* of your environment. You may wonder how people could possibly respect you if you can't even control your bowels.

Since bowel habits generally are not considered an acceptable topic for discussion, you probably have never heard anyone else mention that he or she has trouble controlling his or her bowels. As a result, you may feel that you're the only one with this problem. Many people feel this way. But you should know that *two million people* have fecal incontinence, and each

Recently, major improvements have been made in the management and treatment of incontinence, and technological progress in treatment continues to be made. Knowing that there are medical professionals who can help you, and that treatment is available, may give you the extra incentive you need to seek medical help.

one of them feels alone, too. The truth is, anyone can be incontinent.

Fecal incontinence is a problem that affects people of both sexes, though not equally: more young boys are incontinent than girls, and more young women than young men. It is also more common among young children and elderly people than the rest of the population. As people live longer, fecal incontinence is becoming more prevalent.

About 1 percent of the general population and 30 percent of people in nursing homes have fecal incontinence. In the United States, 1.5 percent of children have difficulty retaining stool; of every four children who have this problem, three are boys. People who have trouble getting around—because they are confined to bed or a wheelchair or because they require a walker or a cane—have the highest incidence of incontinence.

The financial costs of incontinence can be high. At one end of the life span, we find that children who have this problem may be turned away from the public school system. If the problem is severe enough, the school may refuse to keep a child who is incontinent for stool, and then private schooling or home tutoring must be arranged. For elderly people, incontinence is the second most common reason for institutionalization, and nursing homes charge much more for providing the extra care required by a person with this problem.

Fecal incontinence can be a minor nuisance or a terrible tragedy, depending on how severe it is and how you react to it. Reactions of shame, loss of self-esteem, and despair are common when incontinence is severe or chronic, and these reactions may lead to severe depression and social, sexual, and work disability. People who have chronic fecal incontinence beginning in childhood, for example, rarely marry, and more than two-thirds of them never achieve gainful employment. People who develop fecal incontinence as adults often avoid sexual intimacy because they are afraid their partner will be repelled by them. Fear of rejection and fear of being offensive may inhibit people from initiating sexual contact, but their low self-esteem and lack of self-confidence may be the real reason people with fecal incontinence avoid intimacy.

Whether you have only occasional, minor accidents, or whether your problem is more serious, the stigma of fecal incontinence can be so devastating that you may have been unwilling to admit to anyone that you have trouble controlling your bowels. If so, you may have missed the chance to get the help that's available for people with this problem.

Secrecy and denial are common. The spouse of a person with incontinence, for example, may notice stains on underwear or bed linens that the other person ignores. If the spouse asks about it, the other person may deny knowing anything about the stains. Sometimes the parents of a child with incontinence discover soiled clothing hidden in drawers, shoe boxes, or closets. Some people who are incontinent admit only to having a problem with diarrhea, perhaps because diarrhea is considered a more socially acceptable problem.

Because of embarrassment and social shame, you may also avoid telling your physician about a history of incontinence. If you have a condition that can lead to incontinence, and if you and your physician have established a relationship of trust, your physician may discover the problem by carefully and gen-

tly asking you questions. But some physicians are as uncomfortable discussing this problem as their patients are, and the condition very often continues to go undiagnosed and untreated.

It often seems easier to deny that the problem exists, or to keep it a secret from other people, than to discuss it with anyone. But if you can talk about your problem with someone you trust—a spouse, parent, friend, or physician—you may find that that person will put you at ease by listening sympathetically and encouraging you to speak more freely about the problem and how it is affecting you socially and psychologically. This will give you an opportunity to work though your emotional reactions. More importantly, though, the sympathetic listener may give you the encouragement you need to seek professional help. With professional help, many people can entirely overcome their problem, and others can learn to manage the problem so that it no longer affects their lifestyle—or their life. Simply finding out what's *causing* the problem can often make a big difference.

We wrote this book to help the many people who are suffering with fecal incontinence, some of them silently and many of them needlessly. If you are one of these people, we hope that this book will help you understand your problem and the many treatments that are available. We hope that this book will show you how to get started in gaining control. Finally, we hope that the information in these pages will encourage you to find and confide in a medical professional who has the compassion and expertise to help you. This book is not intended to take the place of your doctor.

# CHAPTER TWO

# Understanding How Normal Continence Works

*How Normal Continence Works • The Digestive System • The Mechanical Factors of Continence • The Functional Factors of Continence • The Next Step*

When our body is functioning properly, we can control when and where we defecate. What normally happens is that we sense the need to move our bowels, and then we make a decision about where we will go to do this, and when we will go there. When we receive our body's "signal," we may immediately head to the bathroom, or we may decide to wait a minute, a few minutes, or even longer before making the trip to the bathroom. The term *fecal continence* refers to the ability to retain the contents of the bowels until evacuation becomes convenient.

When fecal continence fails, it is usually because one or more of the factors that maintains continence is not functioning properly. But continence is also dependent upon the exquisite coordination of these factors, so incontinence can also occur if these factors aren't working *together* in a coordinated way. *Fecal incontinence is a signal that something is wrong with the factors that make fecal continence possible.* It's important to remember that fecal incontinence does not *cause* the factors to malfunction. Instead, when these factors malfunction, fecal incontinence can result. Like fever, fecal incontinence is a *symptom*. It is *not* a disease, although it can result from any one of a number of diseases or disorders.

Before looking more closely at the causes of incontinence, it's a good idea to understand the mechanisms that normally help us maintain continence.

## How Normal Continence Works

Normal fecal continence is achieved in the colon (also called the large intestine) and the anus through a system that, in simplest terms, may be compared to a reservoir with a cutoff valve (or pinchcock) at the end. In this model, the reservoir represents the colon, and the anal sphincters are represented by the pinchcock, or cutoff valve, that regulates the flow of material out of the reservoir. In addition to the reservoir and the valve, this system requires some way to sense when the reservoir is full and needs emptying, and some way to signal the cutoff valve when it is the right time to open (to empty the reservoir), and when it must stay closed. In the human body, such signals are passed by nerves to the spinal cord and then up the spinal cord to the brain by the nervous system.

There are four basic mechanisms for maintaining conti-

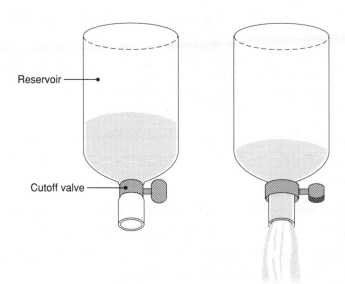

The colon and the anus are like a reservoir with a cutoff valve. The nervous system normally relays messages to the brain about the contents of the reservoir (the colon), and then the brain sends messages to the muscles at the cutoff valve (the anus), telling them either to tighten up (to retain material) or to open up (to permit the evacuation of material).

nence. Of these, the first is the reservoir action of the properly functioning colon, which holds material. The second consists of sensory stimulation and sensory reception. Sensory stimulation takes place when the nerves send a signal to the brain, and sensory reception means that the brain receives the signal from the nerves. The third mechanism is the transmission back down the nervous system of messages (or "orders") from the brain to the muscles, telling them what to do. Fourth is the contraction of the sphincters at the anus (the cutoff valve), which acts to retain material.

To summarize, continence is maintained by these four factors working together:

1. the reservoir action of the colon;
2. the sending and receiving of signals by the nerves to the brain;
3. the sending of signals by the brain to the muscles; and
4. the contraction of the anus in response to signals from the brain.

These four mechanisms can only be effective when the *mechanical* and *functional* factors of continence work together. The anatomical properties of the colon and anus provide the mechanical factors that maintain continence, whereas the functional factors of continence are regulated by the involuntary and voluntary nervous systems. The mechanical factors of continence and the functional factors of continence are interdependent, as we shall see. But even a person with normal anatomy and normal function can have episodes of incontinence, if forces such as urgent, watery diarrhea overwhelm the normal mechanisms.

To better understand these factors and how they are coordinated, it may be helpful to review how the digestive system works. This is a dual purpose system. It's designed to extract liquid and nourishment from the food we eat and to eliminate the waste material that's left over once the liquids and nutrients have been extracted.

## The Digestive System

Food enters the digestive system by way of the lips and mouth. We chew the food and then swallow it down the throat, into the esophagus. Muscles in the walls of the esophagus contract in a stripping wave called *peristalsis,* which moves the food along to the stomach. In the stomach, strong muscles crush the food and mix it with enzymes and acids excreted by the lining of the stomach to help to break the food down.

By the time it leaves the stomach, food has become a watery fluid. This fluid is squeezed into the small intestine, where bile enters from the gallbladder. *Bile,* which breaks down fats in the food, is produced in the liver and then stored in the gallbladder until needed. Other digestive enzymes are also secreted into the intestine by the pancreas gland and the lining of the intestines, and are mixed with the food by the churning movements of the intestinal muscles. As muscles in the walls of the small intestine move the digested material down the intestine (again, by the process of peristalsis), some of this material is absorbed by the lining of the intestine and picked up by blood vessels in the lining. The blood carries this material to various parts of the body. Anything that is not absorbed is emptied from the narrow loops of the small intestine into the wider colon.

Compared to the small intestine, the colon is a sluggish organ, and its peristaltic contractions are less intense than those of the small intestine. So, material normally moves much more slowly through the colon than through the small intestine. The material first moves up the ascending segment of the

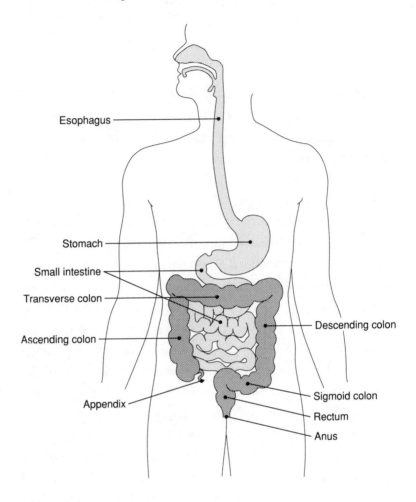

The digestive system.

colon, where much of the water content and many of the minerals are absorbed and the material becomes more solid. As bacteria in the colon continue the process of breaking down the waste material, various substances are released. Sometimes gas is created by this process and may be released through the rectum (flatulence).

At the top of the ascending segment of the colon, the material turns left and enters the transverse segment. As the material travels across the transverse colon, it becomes more formed. (This material, called *feces,* is composed of bacteria, undigested food, and material sloughed from the intestine.) Contractions in the colon next propel the stool down the descending colon, into the S-shaped sigmoid colon and rectum, where it is further dehydrated and stored. The colon and rectum are much more elastic than the small intestine and can therefore hold a large amount of feces prior to defecation.

We can now see how the colon functions as the reservoir in our model, holding stool that gradually becomes more solid as it progresses toward the rectum. The rectum is the lowest part of this reservoir, closest to the opening. In the rectum, a solid column of stool is held ready for elimination.

At the lower end of the rectum is the opening through which feces leave the body. This opening, called the *anus,* is the final inch of the rectum. It is surrounded by the internal anal sphincter except at its very end, where it is surrounded by the external anal sphincter. The anus, composed of the internal and external sphincters, is the cutoff valve in our model. The stool normally is held in the rectum until the act of defecation, when the involuntary and voluntary nervous systems act together to open the internal and external anal sphincters. Then waste material is eliminated through the opening of the anus.

## The Mechanical Factors of Continence

Human anatomy—the way the body is structured—provides several mechanical means of maintaining continence. Bends in the sigmoid colon and in the rectum, for example, act as flap valves to provide one mechanism for mechanical continence. These bends slow the progress of formed stool, and thus they aid in continence. If stool moved more quickly through the colon, we would have great difficulty controlling our bowels, as we sometimes do when diarrhea moves very quickly through the system. When the rectum becomes stretched (or distended) with stool, spiral folds (known as the "valves of Houston") overlap so as to close over each other and hold a column of stool above them. (When the rectum is empty, its lower wall falls into about six longitudinal folds known as the "columns of Morgagni.") The bends or folds help the colon and rectum act as a reservoir for stool.

The rectum also gets some help in maintaining continence from the puborectalis muscle. The puborectalis muscle forms a U-shaped loop, which starts on one side of the rectum and swings behind it and around to the other side. This muscle is normally contracted enough so that it provides a 90-degree angle between the anus and rectum (called the *anorectal angle*). This angle preserves continence, because hard stool does not go around a right angle. When the puborectalis muscle relaxes, however (as it does when we strain to defecate), that 90-degree angle opens up to 130 degrees, and then stool can come down to the anus.

When you're standing up, the anorectal angle becomes

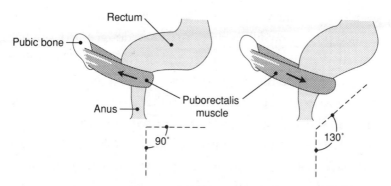

The anorectal angle is provided by the puborectalis muscle. *Left,* the normal 90-degree angle, which helps preserve continence. *Right,* the angle opens up to about 130 degrees when we strain to defecate.

more acute, or shorter or smaller. This helps to counter the effect of gravity on the column of stool, and thus helps preserve continence. Conversely, when you lie down the angle straightens up—but it doesn't matter, because gravity isn't working to bring stool downwards. These folds and angles provide a mechanical mechanism for maintaining continence that conserves energy, because it is effective without any exertion of energy. You don't even have to think about it.

Another mechanical factor that maintains continence is the way the anus is structured. The anus is not round; it is a slit. This slit functions as a *flutter valve.* You can imagine how this works by thinking of a thin, flattened rubber tube. If you blow through the piece of rubber it will flutter, producing a "Bronx cheer" sound. That's exactly what happens when we pass gas: the anus flutters and makes noises.

The anus also preserves continence in the following fashion: when you lift something, or if you laugh, cough, sneeze, or even talk, you increase the pressure on your abdomen. This increased pressure would tend to make you lose control of your bowels if it did not equally compress the anus. The flutter valve works with the bends and folds within the colon and the rectum to even out the pressure so that stool does not escape through the anus as a result of increased pressure on the abdomen. You can see how intricate, how complex, and how coordinated this process is, and how a breakdown of any of its components might result in incontinence.

## The Functional Factors of Continence

Working along with the mechanical factors are the functional factors of continence. While the body's structure is responsible for the mechanical factors, the body's communication system makes the functional factors of continence possible. The nervous systems receive messages about what's going on in the body and send messages telling the body what to do in response.

One of these functional factors of continence involves the inner, or internal, sphincter. In its natural resting state, this muscle is contracted, or closed. It's odd to think of something being *contracted* in its resting state, since we would probably expect something in a resting state to be *relaxed*. Nevertheless, the internal sphincter is contracted in its resting state. It may help to imagine how this works by thinking of a clam as an analogy.

We know that in its natural, resting state, a clam is closed. This is because in its normal state the adductor muscle of a clam is *contracted,* keeping the clam closed. In order for the clam to open up, this muscle must relax. In this way, the internal sphincter is like the adductor muscle of a clam. In its natural state the internal sphincter is constantly closed over, too, and the internal sphincter muscle must relax to allow the anus to open. The internal sphincter is constantly contracted for a reason: contraction prevents the inadvertent loss of liquid material that seeps down in small quantities from the rectum. Most people really don't have to worry, even about small amounts of fairly loose stools: the internal sphincter closes the gates and keeps things from coming out.

When there is enough fecal material to stretch, or distend, the rectum, the internal sphincter will relax reflexively, but only briefly. This momentary relaxation of the internal sphincter sends the signal that the rectum is full and we need to empty our bowels. The internal sphincter opens up for a quick moment, and then it comes back to the resting state. This opening of the internal sphincter is an automatic reflex, like the knee-jerk reflex. We can't inhibit it. This is because the internal sphincter is composed of smooth muscle, which is supplied by nerves from the involuntary nervous system. We have no conscious control over muscles whose nerves come from this system. (Another example of a bodily function that we can't control is peristalsis, which is also performed by smooth muscles.)

This relaxation of the internal sphincter would lead to involuntary loss of stool if we didn't have another functional mechanism for maintaining continence, this one provided by the external sphincter. Unlike the internal sphincter, the external sphincter is composed of striped, or striated, muscle, and therefore it is under the control of the voluntary nervous system. Movement of the external sphincter is generally under our voluntary control, just like the movement of our arms and legs. (A unique feature of the external sphincter is that it is the only striated muscle in the body that is *contracted*—although minimally so—in its natural state. All the other striated muscles in the body—the muscles in the arm, for example—are relaxed in their natural state.)

When the internal sphincter automatically opens in response to distention of the rectum, we rapidly and automatically close the external sphincter even more tightly. We can then voluntarily squeeze even tighter, if we need to. Because we have learned (through toilet training) how to respond appropriately to this stimulus from the internal sphincter, we avoid losing control of our bowels. We "hold" the material back by tightening up on the external sphincter until we are ready to defecate. Contraction of the sphincter muscles also provides part of the pressure that allows the anus to prevent stool from escaping when pressure builds up within the abdomen.

If you think about it, you'll realize that in order to move our bowels, we must overcome the pressure exerted by the anus. We do this by performing something called a *Valsalva maneuver*. In performing a Valsalva maneuver, we close the glottis—close off the airways—and strain, or tighten down, on the abdominal muscles. When we do this, the diaphragm descends like a piston in a cylinder and increases the pressures in the abdomen. If we increase the pressure enough, that inhibits both

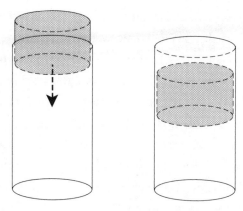

When we bear down to defecate, the diaphragm descends deeper into the abdomen, like a piston (*top*) descends into a cylinder.

the internal sphincter and the external sphincter, and both of them open up and pave the way for evacuation. This is how we exert enough pressure on the anus so that it will open and we can defecate.

If you were designing a system for evacuation of waste products from the body, you probably wouldn't think it was necessary to design such a complex system as this. You would have just one sphincter, and that sphincter would stay closed until you wanted to eliminate waste products, when you would open it. But the reason there are two sphincters is because material has to reach the sensitive nerve endings near the opening of the anus in order for you to get an idea of what's going on down there. This is where the nervous systems come in.

The body's two great nervous systems are the *voluntary nervous system* (also called the *somatic nervous system*) and the *invol-*

*untary nervous system* (also called the *autonomic nervous system*). Much of the voluntary nervous system is cognitive (we think before we act), and much of the involuntary nervous system is reflex (our body reacts to a stimulus without thinking). Both the voluntary and the involuntary nervous systems have branches containing both sensory nerves and motor nerves. Sensory nerves come from parts of the body and go through the spinal cord to the brain—they go up to the brain and give the brain messages about what we feel. Motor nerves come from the brain and go through the spinal cord to muscles—they go down and help the muscles react.

When the rectum is full (and therefore needs to be emptied), motor nerves in the involuntary nervous system cause the internal sphincter to relax momentarily. This permits minute quantities of rectal contents to reach the heavily innervated anal area. The sensory nerves in the involuntary nervous system pick up the message and send it to the brain. In response to this message, motor nerves in the voluntary nervous system cause the external sphincter to contract, and thus continence is maintained until it is convenient for the person to move his or her bowels.

The sensory nerves in the mucosa, or lining, of the rectum (and for that matter in the rest of the gut) really can't appreciate any sensation other than stretch. You can pinch the colon from the inside, scratch it, or even burn it, and it can't feel that—it only feels stretch. But as you get closer to the end of the rectum (toward the anus), the covering is more like skin. In this area, there is a profusion of different nerve endings that are extremely sensitive to touch, pressure, and temperature—

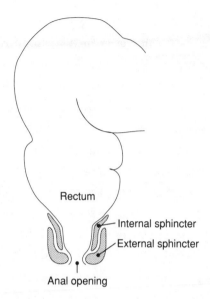

Rectum

Internal sphincter

External sphincter

Anal opening

When the internal sphincter relaxes, the external sphincter contracts in response.

are sensitive enough, in other words, to determine what the physical state of matter is, whether it is solid, liquid, or gas.

So what happens is, during that momentary reflex relaxation of the internal sphincter, that slit opens and minute quantities of fecal material come down and touch those sensitive nerve endings in the external sphincter just long enough for the "sampling reflex" to take place. Once the material is sampled, a message goes up to the brain as to whether you're dealing with solids, liquids, or gases. And once you become aware of that, then you can take appropriate action: you can either tighten up and prevent the material from going farther, or you can go to the bathroom. The sensory nerves (which sense what's going on and send messages up the spinal cord to the brain) and the motor nerves (which create movement) act together to coordinate continence.

Continence is even more complicated than this, however. In the chain of events described above, the brain has to be able to sense what's going on before you can take voluntary action. But things happen so fast during the momentary relaxation of the internal sphincter that you can't wait for the brain to get that message. For this reason, the external sphincter has to respond automatically in order to preserve continence. Contracting the external sphincter in response to the stimulus that reflexively relaxes the internal sphincter is so well learned early in life that it becomes an automatic response. For this reason, it is considered a *learned automatic response*. Even though it is still within our voluntary control, closing the external sphincter in response to the stimulus that reflexively relaxes the internal sphincter is something we usually do without thinking.

These are all parts of how we maintain continence. It is easy to understand how continence might be affected if any of these factors fail, or if they fail to work together in a coordinated way. But so far we've only considered the retentive forces involved in continence. There are aggressive forces that move material through the colon, too. Think about how much easier it is to retain solid material than it is to retain urgent diarrhea or liquid material. When the normal functioning of the colon is upset for any reason (such as when you have the stomach flu) and the stool does not harden in the normal way, liquid material may be propelled through urgent contractions of the colon. Under certain circumstances, even the strongest sphincter muscles may not be able to hold back severe diarrhea.

## The Next Step

Understanding how normal continence works will probably help you understand what's interfering with your normal bowel function. Once you've made the decision to find out what's causing your problem, it's time to take the next step and consult with your doctor. Your doctor will take a medical history, perform a physical examination, and probably do some tests. He or she may also refer you to a specialist—for example, a gastroenterologist (a doctor who specializes in diagnosing and treating disorders of the digestive system) or a surgeon. The doctor has to determine what's causing your incontinence before he or she can help you, because the treatment for fecal incontinence depends on the cause. Finding out what's causing your incontinence is what the next two chapters are about.

# CHAPTER THREE

# Finding Out the Cause of Your Problem

*Keeping a Symptom Diary* · *Visiting the Doctor* ·
*The Medical History* · *The Physical Examination*

The first step in gaining control is to find out where and why normal continence is breaking down—to discover what's interfering with your normal bowel function. That's what we want to do in this chapter. We want to concentrate on *finding out* the cause of your incontinence. Your doctor will play an important role in helping to discover the cause of the problem. Before you visit your doctor, though, it's a good idea to keep a symptom diary. For this reason, we'll lead off this chapter by describing how you might go about keeping such a diary.

## Keeping a Symptom Diary

The symptom diary is a simple device for keeping track of accidents. The diary is a written record of episodes of fecal incontinence. We recommend that you keep such a diary for one or two weeks before you go to the doctor. The symptom diary will give your doctor some of the information that he or she needs in order to make an accurate diagnosis. Your doctor will probably ask you to keep the diary during some stages of treatment, too, so you both can keep track of your progress.

It's not hard to keep a symptom diary. The way it works is this: Whenever you have a bowel movement of any kind, write down a complete description of it. We recommend that you keep your diary in a separate notebook. (It doesn't seem to work very well to keep your symptom diary in the same place you keep track of appointments or other things to do.) In the notebook, you might want to set up columns like the ones in the sample symptom diary reproduced on page 27. The columns help you remember to record all the important information. If you have an accident, you'll need to record when and where it happened, how serious it was, what else was going on in your life when the accident happened, how you responded emotionally to the accident, and how the accident affected your lifestyle.

Begin with the easiest information: Every time you have a bowel movement, whether intentionally or accidentally, write down the day and the time of day. This information will help both you and your doctor develop an accurate picture of how often you have accidents and when your accidents are most likely to occur (if you have a pattern of accidents, that is— some people don't). If there's a difference between weekends and weekdays, for example, there may be something about your weekend or weekday lifestyle that's affecting your control.

If you have an accident, describe the accident. Where did it happen? Were you awake or asleep when it happened? Was the stool liquid, loose, or solid? Were you passing gas when it happened? Was there enough fecal material just to soil your underwear slightly, or to soil it heavily? Or did you have a "major accident"? Did you have a warning before the accident occurred, or did you become aware of it only while it was happening or after it happened? This information, combined with information about the frequency of accidents, will give both you and your doctor an indication of how severe your problem is.

Then write down what you were doing when you had the accident, what you ate before the accident, whether you were alone or someone was with you. Write down everything and anything that might be relevant. This information may provide the first clue about the cause of your problem, by revealing how your daily schedule, your diet, your activities, and your daily life events are related to your accidents.

Finally, write how each accident affected you—whether you reacted to the accident by changing your plans, for example. Did you leave an important meeting? Did you decide to stay home instead of going out, as you had planned? By relaying this information, the diary will let you and your doctor know what effect accidents have on your life and your well-being. It will tell you how incontinence is affecting your quality of life. Be sure to write down how your accident affects the lives of the people who are closest to you, too. Their reactions influence your emotional and social well-being.

If you have been incontinent for a long time, you may already know what your pattern of incontinence is like. It may

# SYMPTOM DIARY

| Date and time of normal bowel movement | Date and time of accident | Description of accident: solid, liquid, or gas? small or large amount? any warning? | Food, activities, stress, and other factors the day of the accident | How you reacted and how others reacted |
|---|---|---|---|---|
| | | | | |
| | | | | |
| | | | | |
| | | | | |
| | | | | |
| | | | | |
| | | | | |
| | | | | |
| | | | | |
| | | | | |
| | | | | |
| | | | | |
| | | | | |
| | | | | |
| | | | | |
| | | | | |

be that, for you, passage of a small amount of liquid stool while you sleep is a fairly regular occurrence and has been for some time. In that case, you may feel it's unnecessary to keep a symptom diary before seeing the doctor. But we encourage you to begin the habit of keeping a symptom diary, anyway. For one thing, your doctor will probably ask you to keep a diary once treatment starts. But it's also worth considering that people who think they know exactly when and where (and why) accidents occur are sometimes surprised by what they find out when they keep a written record.

## Visiting the Doctor

Some people see the doctor about incontinence because they are staining and they are embarrassed about it. Other people go because they are worried about what the incontinence means—they're worried that it might mean there's something seriously wrong with them. Whatever the reason they decide to seek medical help, most people begin with their family physician, because they know him or her and feel more comfortable talking with the family physician than they would with a stranger. But some people are *more* comfortable talking about this subject with a doctor they don't know, and they would prefer to keep the family physician for routine matters like checkups and sore throats. This is okay, too, but your family physician should at least be made aware of the problem.

You can find a doctor who is a specialist in this area by asking your family physician to recommend one, or if you regularly see a gynecologist (a doctor specializing in women's health) or a urologist (a specialist in the treatment of urinary problems), you can ask that person to refer you to an internist or a gastroenterologist. (An internist is a doctor specializing in the diagnosis and nonsurgical treatment of diseases; a gastroenterologist, as we noted earlier, is a doctor who specializes in the diagnosis and treatment of disorders of the digestive system.) The city or state medical society and some hospitals will refer you to a doctor if you call up and ask. Be sure to tell them what the problem is, so they can refer you to the best doctor for this problem. Or you might ask your friends for the name of their doctor.

We acknowledge that when you visit the doctor, he or she will ask questions that may make you feel awkward or embarrassed. For the *doctor,* however, these questions are routine, and you don't have to feel embarrassed because of what you may think the doctor is thinking about what you're saying. Your doctor *wants* to find out what the problem is, and he or she has to ask you these questions to do that.

When it comes to answering these questions, it may help to think of your doctor as a mechanic trying to find out what's wrong with the motor in a car. Your doctor knows all about the digestive system and bowel habits and approaches a problem in this area the same way he or she approaches a problem in the circulatory system or the reproductive system. If you feel uncomfortable with your doctor, however, or (perhaps more importantly) if you feel that your doctor is uncomfortable discussing this area of your body with you, you might want to consult a different doctor.

If you want to, you can take a spouse, partner, or friend along with you when you visit the doctor. You should go with someone or go alone, depending on what makes you comfortable. Spouses and live-in friends sometimes go to the doctor with the patient and talk about how they're managing this problem in their life. That is usually best, but it's up to you.

## The Medical History

When you visit your doctor, the first thing he or she will do is ask you a lot of questions. This is called taking the medical history. The medical history tells the doctor what your symptoms are and how they're affecting you and your quality of life. It also tells the doctor what effect the incontinence is having on your family. Sometimes the medical history reveals an underlying medical condition that may be causing or contributing to your incontinence.

Many people find it easier to answer their doctor's questions if they keep a symptom diary for one or two weeks before the appointment (see the description of this diary, above). Take the symptom diary to the doctor's office with you. Having an accurate, written record of when and where accidents occur will give your doctor a head start on finding out the cause of your problem. Also, your doctor can refer to your diary entries while he or she asks you questions. By giving you and your doctor a place to start, the symptom diary may help put both of you at ease.

The doctor's role in taking the medical history is to ask you questions that will lead you to give the doctor the information he or she needs to make an initial diagnosis. Performing this role effectively involves making the patient feel comfortable. Doctors are trained in how to do this, but some doctors are better at it than others. If you are uncomfortable, there's a chance you won't get the full benefit of treatment. Unless you feel comfortable, you may not answer your doctor's questions honestly or completely. This is very important. You should not withhold information from your doctor, because you may be withholding exactly the piece of information he or she needs to make a diagnosis and determine proper treatment. Discuss your discomfort with your doctor. Again, if the problem is with the doctor or your relationship with the doctor, it may be worth going to a different doctor who may be better skilled at putting patients at ease.

When they are seeing a patient for the first time for incontinence, many doctors ask the patient to complete a questionnaire. Like the symptom diary, the questionnaire gives the doctor a place to start. Also, the questionnaire sometimes indicates that there's a difference between the patient's perception of the problem and the patient's ability to tolerate the problem. That is, the problem may not be as bad as the patient thinks it is, or it may be worse than the patient thinks it is. The questionnaire sometimes helps the patient and the doctor understand just exactly how severe the problem is.

Whether your doctor uses a questionnaire or just asks you questions orally, he or she is looking for the same kind of information. The doctor will probably begin by asking you questions related to the state of your incontinence. We'll consider this the first half of the medical history.

Often, the first question the doctor asks is how old you were when incontinence began (this is called *age at onset*). If you've had incontinence since you were born, the incontinence may be caused by a congenital problem (a problem that was present when you were born). If the incontinence began during toilet training, or after a period of psychological stress, it's possible that the incontinence is functional (related to behavior). A person who was never incontinent and then has several accidents may have either a medical condition that's causing incontinence or a fecal impaction of the bowel which is interfering with normal defecation (fecal impactions are discussed in Chapter 7).

How long you've had the problem—the *duration* of incontinence—can be calculated from the age of onset to the present. In addition to the duration of incontinence, the doctor will want to know your *pattern* of incontinence. To find out, he or she will ask you whether you have occasional accidents (*episodic incontinence*) or regular accidents (*continuous incontinence*). The doctor will also ask you whether the problem has stayed the same (*static incontinence*) or has gotten worse (*progressive incontinence*). The duration and pattern of incontinence can be very revealing. A person who has always had normally formed stools but who suddenly is unable to control the passage of liquid stool may have an acute illness accompanied by diarrhea, for example.

Next, the doctor will ask you questions designed to uncover the *degree* of fecal incontinence (whether mild, moderate, or severe), its *nature* (solid, liquid, or gas),* and its *frequency*. You can get a good idea of the frequency of incontinence by keeping track of how many accidents you have during a day and how often you need to change your bed linens, underclothes, or pads. The symptom diary can be helpful here.

To understand your *degree of control,* your doctor will ask you how long you can maintain continence after you experience a strong urge to defecate. Can you delay evacuation for a minute or more, less than a minute, or not at all? Can you delay evacuation of solid stool better than you can delay evacuation of liquid stool or gas? The doctor will want to know about any special circumstances that result in an episode of incontinence. For example, does physical activity make you have an accident? Incontinence brought on by physical activity is called "stress incontinence."

In taking the medical history, the doctor will want to become familiar with your *bowel habits.* He or she will ask whether you are generally constipated before you have an episode of incontinence or whether, conversely, your accidents usually occur when you have diarrhea. Your doctor will want to know how many bowel movements you usually have during a day (1 or 2? 3 to 5? more than 5?), or whether you don't have a bowel movement every day. He or she will also ask about the consistency of the stool (whether it is solid, loose, or liquid). Information about bowel habits can provide important diagnostic clues.

---

*People can be incontinent for solids, liquids, or gas, or for a combination of these. Also, liquid stool or small quantities of solids can inadvertently be lost during the passage of gas.

Do you have to strain to defecate and, if so, how long have you had to do this? Do you ever have blood in your stool? Do you have abdominal cramps before or during defecation? Your doctor will want to know whether, once you have moved your bowels, you never, sometimes, or always feel as if you haven't completely emptied your bowels. Do you sometimes feel as if there is more material there, but you can't get it out?

Your degree of *sensory awareness* about the urge to defecate can influence how much control you have over your bowels. The first aspect of sensory awareness has to do with whether you receive your body's message loud and clear when you have the urge to defecate. Do you strongly feel it when you need to defecate, or are you uncertain what you're feeling, or whether you're feeling the urge at all? Or do you seldom or never feel the urge to defecate? Sensory awareness also involves being able to distinguish between solid, liquid, and gas. When you receive your body's signal, can you always, sometimes, or never tell whether you have to pass solid stool, liquid stool, or gas?

Since lifestyle factors can influence continence, the doctor will ask about your diet. Have you noticed that certain foods cause you to pass gas more than usual or affect the frequency or nature of your bowel movements? Are there any foods that you avoid because you suspect they give you trouble? Milk products are a frequent source of digestive problems in people who cannot tolerate lactose (this is called *lactose intolerance*). The doctor will also want to know about any recent trips you have taken or any recent changes you have made in your lifestyle. Have you moved to a new home, for example, or has your schedule changed at work? The doctor may ask you about any history of anal sex or anal manipulation or injury, since this can affect the tone of the muscles in the anus. The doctor will certainly ask you about any medications you are taking, since many medications can interfere with muscular or central nervous system functioning.

To complete the first half of the medical history—the actual state of incontinence—the doctor will ask you about your quality of life. He or she will want to know whether incontinence interferes with your daily activities or only interferes with some social activities. And what about your family and friends? Their reaction to your incontinence can tell the doctor a great deal about the severity of your problem and how the problem is affecting your life.

In taking the second half of your medical history, the doctor will be looking for information about associated conditions you may have that can contribute to incontinence. He or she will ask you whether you have ever been told that you have one of a number of conditions. These include neurological disorders such as spinal cord lesions, gastrointestinal disorders such as irritable bowel syndrome, and systemic disorders such as neuromuscular and connective tissue diseases. Local anal disease is another condition associated with incontinence. It can impair sphincter function, but it can also be mistaken for fecal incontinence because it produces a discharge that drains from the anus. Finally, the doctor will ask you whether you have experienced certain medical events that can contribute to incontinence. For example, if you are a woman with fecal incontinence, the doctor may ask you whether you have had an obstetrical injury such as a delivery tear in the perineal area. A history of prolonged labor, forceps delivery, difficulty evacuating the bowels after giving birth, or incontinence following childbirth may also reveal the origin of your problem.

The doctor will ask, have you ever had any spinal disorder or back injury? radiotherapy? bladder, uterine, rectal, or anal prolapse? anorectal or intestinal surgery? Injury that occurs during hemorrhoid surgery or a fissure operation can impair the sphincters or the nerves to the sphincters, as can an industrial accident or an automobile accident. The doctor will want to distinguish between injury to the sphincter muscle and injury to nerves, since treatment for them is different.

A summary of the medical history is presented below. (Medical conditions and other factors that can contribute to incontinence are discussed in chapters 5 and 7.)

### MEDICAL HISTORY FOR FECAL INCONTINENCE

### The State of Incontinence

1. Age at onset
2. Duration
3. Pattern (episodic or continuous, static or progressive)
4. Degree (mild, moderate, severe)
5. Nature (solid, liquid, gas)
6. Frequency
7. Degree of control
8. Bowel habits (including straining)
9. Sensory awareness

10. Lifestyle factors, including medications
11. Quality of life

### Associated Conditions and Medical Events

1. Associated conditions (central nervous system and spinal cord impairment, systemic disorders, and local disorders)
2. Medical events (delivery history; history of anal trauma)

## *The Physical Examination*

Once he or she has made a preliminary diagnosis of the cause of your incontinence based on the medical history, your doctor will examine you. The physical examination may begin with a thorough neurological examination, to find out if you have any nerve problems (like a person who has had a stroke might have). As we have seen, if the nerves that communicate the body's message about the need to defecate are impaired, control can be affected. The doctor will tap your knees with a rubber mallet and will check your arms and legs for strength and sensory perception.

In examining you, the doctor will also look for any systemic disorders that can cause incontinence, such as hyperthyroidism, which can cause impairment of many muscles, including the sphincter muscles. The doctor will check for postural hypotension (a sudden drop in blood pressure when the person stands upright), which is a condition that can be associated with diabetes and can impair the involuntary nervous system serving the gut. People with diabetes often have diarrhea, especially nocturnal diarrhea, and are more vulnerable to incontinence while they're sleeping. The physical examination should also detect neuromuscular disorders such as multiple sclerosis and the muscular dystrophies.

Next comes examination of the anal area, which is very important in making the initial diagnosis. Many people are uncomfortable with the whole idea of this part of the examination. Some people avoid going to the doctor because they are embarrassed at the thought of having a rectal examination, or because they've heard that it hurts. Many causes of incontinence can only be detected by a rectal examination, however.

Because women have internal examinations for gynecological care, they may be somewhat more used to the idea than men. Men above the age of 50 are also more likely to be accustomed to a rectal examination, since that examination needs to be done annually after the age of 50, to check the prostate gland for enlargement. Many people need extra reassurance from their partner or from the doctor, however. Again, it may help to keep in mind that your doctor is a professional who has done this many times before.

This very necessary and very important part of the physical examination includes visual inspection, a pinprick test, and digital (finger) examination of the anal area. The digital rectal examination is simple and takes only a few seconds. It may be uncomfortable, but it seldom hurts, and it is over quickly.

To make a reliable diagnosis, the doctor needs to inspect your underclothes and the perianal area (the area around the anus), to see for himself or herself what the soiling is like. This visual inspection allows the doctor to get a better idea of the degree and nature of the soiling—whether it is stool, blood, or mucus. It also lets the doctor know whether the soiling has broken down the skin in the area (this process is called *maceration*). The doctor will be able to detect any scars, too, such as a scar from an episiotomy. A scar of any kind may indicate that the area has been injured in the past, and can provide a significant clue for diagnosis, since people sometimes don't know or don't remember that they've been injured and so don't report the injury in the medical history. Lopsidedness (or asymmetry) of the anal area may also provide a clue about previous scarring and trauma, perhaps from anal surgery performed in the past.

When the buttocks are spread, the doctor will look to see whether the anus is closed, as it should be, or gaping, which indicates a problem with muscle tone. The doctor will check the anus for crevices or other defects that can allow liquid stool to leak out. The doctor will note the position of the anus, since anal displacement may indicate a congenital problem. Finally, the doctor will ask you to contract your anus voluntarily (tighten your sphincters) and will note whether the anus puckers (as it should) when you squeeze.

The doctor will test the anal wink reflex with a light pinprick and touch test in four quadrants of the anus (upper left, upper right, lower right, lower left). If the nerves and muscles are intact, the anus will respond to a pin scratch in the anal area with a wink reflex (it will close up tighter). This reflex may be missing, or it may be difficult to elicit this reflex, in someone with a neuropathy (impaired function of the nerves). (Neuropathy and other causes of fecal incontinence are described in Chapter 5.) By testing each of the four quadrants, the doctor can locate the site of the weakness, if there is any.

In the digital examination, the doctor gently slides a gloved, lubricated finger into the rectum. By properly performing the digital rectal examination, the doctor can find out many things. First, whether the stretched anus is smooth, as it should be, or roughened and irregular. Roughness inside the anus indicates that the person might have a fissure, or a tear in the walls of the anus. An irregular surface suggests that the person might have some scars in the region. The doctor will ask you to tighten the sphincters again, this time so that their strength can be assessed. Be sure to tell your doctor if the finger examination is painful, because that would provide evidence that you have a fissure, an abscess, or a perianal excoriation (an injury in which the skin has been scraped).

The doctor can also determine whether the resting tone of the anal canal is normal or increased or decreased, and to what degree. Remember that the internal sphincter is naturally *contracted* in its resting state. About 70 percent of the resting tone of the anal canal is provided by the internal sphincter, the rest being provided by the external sphincter. Digital examination provides a rough estimate of the tone in the canal, so the doctor has an idea of whether your problem might be related to an improperly functioning sphincter. A loss of sphincter control can result from a muscular problem or a neurological problem, or it may be related to local anal disease. The doctor will be able to detect any mass of hard stool in the rectum; such a mass can be a sign of a fecal impaction.

The doctor will bend the examining finger toward the coccyx (tailbone), to see whether the anus opens wider in response. Such a response, called a *gaping reflex,* can be a sign of neurological impairment. With the finger in this position, the doctor can also measure the angle between the anus and the posterior (rear) wall of the rectum. As we have seen, when the puborectalis muscle is intact and functioning properly, the angle between the anus and the rectum measures roughly 90 degrees. If the doctor determines that the angle is greater than 90 degrees, he or she may suspect that you have a prolapse or an internal intussusception (a condition in which one part of the intestine is pushed into another part of the intestine). While the finger is still in this position, the doctor will ask you to contract the sphincter. When everything is functioning properly, the doctor will be able to feel the puborectalis muscle pulling the examining finger forward as you squeeze.

Next, if you are a woman, the doctor will turn the finger around, pointing it toward the front of the rectum. By doing this, the doctor can tell whether you might have a rectocele (a protrusion of part of the wall of the rectum into the vagina). If a rectocele is detected, the doctor will be able to tell how large it is. A rectocele may result when a woman gives birth in a difficult delivery, but symptoms of a rectocele may not show up for fifteen or twenty years after the delivery. When the digital examination is nearly over, the doctor may insert another finger into the vagina, to determine how thick the rectovaginal septum and the perineal body are. Hernias, tumors, and inflammation can be detected in this way.

At the conclusion of the examination, the doctor will slowly withdraw the finger out of the anus. While doing this, the doctor will ask you to contract the sphincter so he or she can check how strongly you can contract the external sphincter on command. Although only 30 percent of the *resting* tone of the anal canal is provided by the external sphincter, when the patient's muscles are contracted, the external sphincter ought to have a strong response, because most of the *contracted* tone of the anal canal is provided by the external sphincter.

Your doctor may be able to make a preliminary diagnosis based on the information he or she has gathered from the medical history and the physical examination. It's often a good idea to confirm this diagnosis with diagnostic tests, which can also uncover findings that have been missed in the history or the physical examination. The tests used to diagnose the cause of fecal incontinence are described in the next chapter. Your doctor may ask you to have some of these tests.

# CHAPTER FOUR

# Diagnostic Tests

*Proctoscopy, Sigmoidoscopy, and Anoscopy* ·
*Barium Enema or Colonoscopy* · *Colon Motility*
*Studies* · *Electromyography* · *Defecography* ·
*Anorectal Ultrasound* · *Rectal Saline Infusion Test*

Sometimes there is still uncertainty about the diagnosis, even after the doctor has taken a medical history and performed a physical examination, and then tests are ordered to help identify the cause of the problem. Sometimes diagnostic tests are performed so the doctor can get a better idea of the severity of the problem and have a basis for future follow-up. If you are being treated for fecal incontinence, your doctor may also ask you to have one or more tests so both you and the doctor can monitor your progress.

The following tests are the ones most commonly performed to identify the cause and severity of fecal incontinence, and to monitor progress during treatment. The tests are described here in the order in which they are usually performed, beginning with the tests that are done most often. Tests are usually performed in a doctor's office or in the outpatient setting of a hospital. The person who conducts the test may be a doctor, a nurse, or a trained technician but will almost certainly be someone who is highly skilled in these kinds of tests.

If while you are having a test done you feel very uncomfortable or feel any pain, it is important to say so. Most of the tests are not painful (we tell you which ones are), but you should say something if you feel pain, anyway. The person performing the test may be able to do something to make you more comfortable, may change the approach of the test, or may stop the test altogether. Or the person can tell you how much longer the test will take and may reassure you that the discomfort you're feeling is a normal response to the test.

## *Proctoscopy, Sigmoidoscopy, and Anoscopy*

Depending on where he or she thinks your problem is, your doctor may want to look inside your anus, rectum, or sigmoid colon. While you lie on your side, the doctor will use an instrument called a *scope* to look inside. The scope may be either a rigid tube with a light on it or a flexible fiber optic tube that can be bent. Through the scope, the doctor can see signs of fissures, hemorrhoids, or inflammation in the anus, or inflammation or tumors in the rectum and colon. (The anus, remember, is the final inch of the rectum, the rectum is above the anus, and the sigmoid colon is right above the rectum.) An anoscopy is the test for looking inside the anus, the proctoscopy looks at the rectum (*procto* means *rectum*), and the sigmoidoscopy looks at the sigmoid colon. The proctosigmoidoscopy looks at both the rectum and the sigmoid. Depending on the test, an anoscope, proctoscope, or sigmoidoscope is used.

## Barium Enema or Colonoscopy

After the proctosigmoidoscopy, in some instances the doctor may decide that there's a need to know more about the remaining part of the colon, above the sigmoid, and may want to perform either a colonoscopy or a barium enema. The colonoscopy is like a sigmoidoscopy except that the scope is a longer flexible instrument that can be inserted into the entire colon. Since this scope can go much higher, the doctor can visualize the entire colon.

The colonscopy causes discomfort, so before the test the patient is usually given an injection of a medication similar to Valium along with a pain killer. This creates a mild sedation called conscious sedation or "twilight sleep." In conscious sedation the person doesn't lose consciousness but is in a very relaxed state. This test is not often necessary for problems of incontinence.

The barium enema is an x-ray study in which barium—a white, pasty material—is inserted into the rectum while the patient is lying on his or her side on an x-ray table. Then x-rays are taken and interpreted by a specially trained physician called a radiologist. Since x-rays don't go through barium (it is radio-opaque), the barium appears as a shadow on the x-ray film.

The x-rays outline the colon and the rectum and allow the doctor to see structures that we don't normally see.

This study is not always needed and is used at the discretion of the examining physician. It can produce pain like gas pain as the colon is distended with barium. After the test the patient is sent to the bathroom to get rid of the barium. Any pain that may be present usually subsides when the barium is expelled. Because it involves the use of x-rays, the barium enema is to be avoided by pregnant women and women who have any chance of being pregnant.

The evening *before* having a barium enema, the patient will use laxatives at home, as instructed by the doctor's office. Once the patient's system has been cleaned out with laxatives, the patient must keep the system empty by not eating anything until after the test.

## Colon Motility Studies

This is a general term for any kind of study that measures pressures within the colon. Colon motility studies really consist of a series of tests that are performed all at one time. They can only be performed by a person who is skilled in giving these tests and in using the testing equipment.

As we saw in Chapter 2, fecal incontinence can be caused by nerve problems or by muscle problems, or both. Motility tests can determine whether the nerves or the muscles are impaired. Some people have very good sensation (they have intact sensory nerves) and good motor nerves, but they may not be able to squeeze well because they have muscle problems. That is, the sensory nerves to the spine and up to the brain, and the motor nerves back down the spine to the muscle, are intact, but the muscle is weak or isn't functioning because of infection, abscesses, fissures—or because of surgery performed to try to correct some of these things (see Chapter 5). The nerves give the right message to the muscle, but the muscle either responds too weakly to preserve continence or doesn't respond at all.

Other people have a nerve problem that affects, say, the sensory nerves only, so they don't sense when they need to squeeze down. The motor nerves to the muscle are intact, and the muscle is intact, and they can voluntarily make it squeeze down, but the reflex doesn't occur—they don't sense the need to defecate as it is signaled by the distention of the rectum. For these people, the muscle function is fine, and they can make the squeeze needed to preserve continence, but they don't sense when they need to do so.

Others may have normal sensory function and normal muscles, but their motor nerves are impaired. For them, sensation is normal—they *feel* the distention of the rectum—and the muscles could respond properly to a signal from the motor nerves, but the motor nerves can't signal the muscles to respond.

In colon motility studies, muscle function is tested by inserting small balloons into the sphincters and the rectum. A small balloon is used in the rectum, and then two even smaller air-filled balloons are used, one in the internal sphincter and one in the external sphincter. The rectal balloon is inflated (filled with air) to mimic collection of stool in rectum, so the test reveals how the sphincters and the rectum function in response to this stimulus. Remember that when stool enters the rectum and distends the walls, the internal sphincter opens reflexively, and the external sphincter closes up at the same time the internal sphincter opens. When a colon motility study is performed, the doctor or technician will inflate the balloons and then observe how the patient's rectum and sphincters respond.

The response of the rectum and the sphincters to the inflation of the rectal balloon is measured by pressure transducers. Each of the three balloons is attached to a pressure transducer, and each pressure transducer sends a signal that is picked up by a polygraph, which records the signal by means of pens that write on graph paper that continuously unrolls beneath the recording pens. In this way this test is like an electrocardiogram, another test in which pens write on graph paper to record measurements from inside the body. (In an electrocardiogram, the electrical activity of the heart is measured and recorded by the tracing pens.)

In one kind of colon motility study, called an *anorectal motility study,* there are three recording pens: one records the pressure in the rectum, one the pressure in the internal sphincter, and one the pressure in the external sphincter. When the muscles contract, the pressure in the balloons changes, and these pressure changes are transmitted to the pressure transducers, which convert them to electrical signals that can be picked up by the recording pens on the polygraph.

Colon motility tests include recordings of sphincter and colon motility. The term *colon motility study* can be confusing because, unfortunately, it is used to describe the combination of the two (anal sphincter studies and colon motility studies) as well as the colon motility study by itself. Your doctor may call these *manometric tests* or *manometry*, which simply means "measuring pressures."

*Anal sphincter studies* (also called anal rectal manometry) involve measuring the resting pressure of the sphincter muscles and the changes in those pressures during reflex responses that are stimulated by the rectal distention caused by inflation of the balloons. You will be asked to squeeze the sphincters at various times during the testing, so that the function of your muscles and nerves can be assessed. The muscles of the colon are assessed at the same time as the muscles of the sphincter.

In the colon motility study, what's studied is colonic accommodation (the elasticity or compliance of the colon) and the contractions of the muscles of the colon. To measure colonic motility, the technician first finds out what's going on in the basal state (when the colon is resting). Then, by filling the balloon gradually with air, the technician and the physician find out how the colon adapts to a buildup of material in it. As we saw in Chapter 2, as stool gradually builds up, the colon has to be elastic, and has to dilate elastically as a reservoir, to accommodate the stool. The colonic motility study finds out what volume the rectum can tolerate or contain before it goes into spasm to move things out. With inflammation (proctitis or colitis), the volume is very small—the rectum loses its elasticity and doesn't have a good reservoir capacity. It goes into spasm (as recorded on the graph paper) at low levels of distention. Sometimes the problem is that the colon is *too* elastic, and it keeps expanding and expanding, without reacting to the buildup of material by squeezing to move it out. (This condition, called *megacolon,* is discussed in Chapter 7.)

*The rectal sensitivity test* is done as part of these studies. During the tests, the technician will ask the patient to answer questions about what he or she is feeling. The patient is asked to report sensations because the doctor and the technician are interested in learning at what level the patient can begin to feel certain things. They know the threshold—the pressure at which a person *ought* to begin to feel—and they can compare that threshold with what the patient is telling them. The person may have sensation, but large volumes of air and huge pressure may be required before that sensation is appreciated. By monitoring the input of air and the patient's verbal description of sensation, the technician and the doctor can tell a great deal about the person's sensory abilities in this area. (This technique can also measure a person's response to treatment such as biofeedback, to find out whether that treatment brings abnormal response levels down, closer to the normal threshold. See Chapter 6.)

## Electromyography

In this test, electromyographic signals (the electrical signals that the muscles put out) are assessed to determine how tightly the patient can squeeze the sphincters. The doctor or technician prepares the patient for this test either by pasting electrodes on the buttocks over the sphincter or by inserting into the rectum a small finger-shaped probe with electrodes on the sides of it. When a nerve stimulates the muscles, the muscles release electrical currents. The electrodes pick up changes in electrical activity in the muscles and measure the electrical activity that the muscles put out.

An instrument called a perineometer is often used to display the signals that are picked up by the electrodes. Multicolored lights in a circle or ring on the face of the instrument represent the sphincter itself. The perineometer provides a visual display of the patient's response. The stronger the response, the more lights are lit up. This is a different way of displaying the information that is displayed by the recording pens in the polygraph, described above. This test is similar to biofeedback techniques, in which electrodes may be placed over the forehead muscle, or any muscle in the body, to pick up muscle activity and measure muscle strength there.

The anal plug that is sometimes used in these tests can also be used to check the four quadrants of the anus. It can pick up a localized defect in the sphincter, such as a scar (see Chapter 5), because if there is a defect in a specific part of the sphincter, the lights corresponding to that part of the sphincter won't light up.

## Defecography

This test, also called *proctography,* is done in order to visualize the lower part of the intestines, the rectum, and the sphincters. It is used more often than the barium enema to investigate fecal incontinence, and it is similar to a barium enema. A difference is that in defecography, only a small amount of barium is used and the patient is sitting on a stool rather than lying down. Unlike with the barium enema, no clean-out preparation or fasting is required. An x-ray tube takes pictures from the side as the patient sits on a stool. With this test the doctor wants to see what the muscles are doing as the patient is tightening muscles or straining to defecate, so the barium comes out during the test.

Under normal circumstances, certain muscle groups (called agonists) ought to contract and other muscle groups (antagonists) ought to relax when a person bears down to evacuate. When these things happen, the anorectal angle—the angle at which the rectum meets the anus—changes. We know that the anorectal angle ought to change from 90 degrees (its normal resting angle) to 130 degrees during attempts to defecate. X-rays taken during this test will reveal the anorectal angle and thereby indicate whether the puborectalis muscle is functioning properly.

During the test the patient is asked to tighten the muscles, and subsequently to strain down. As the patient does this, x-ray images are taken of the barium moving through the rectum and sphincters. Any muscle weaknesses, internal hernias (rectoceles), or internal prolapses can be detected. Because it involves the use of x-rays, the defecography is to be avoided by pregnant women and women who have any chance of being pregnant.

## Anorectal Ultrasound

Ultrasound works by sending out a sound signal. (It is not an x-ray.) When the sound bounces back it is picked up, and the object that the sound is bouncing off of can be outlined. Ultrasound is often used to pick up the outline of a submarine or fish under water. In anorectal ultrasound, the objects being outlined are the muscles of the anus.

In anorectal ultrasound (also called *sonography*), a probe shaped like a finger is inserted into the anal canal and rectum. That probe has a spinning wheel inside it that sends out a sound signal in a circular fashion. When the sound bounces back, all of the muscles surrounding the rectum and the anal canal can be seen on a video screen. On the screen you can see the muscles at rest and you can see the muscles moving, just like you can see the baby moving inside the mother's womb during fetal ultrasound testing. This test allows the doctor to see how the muscles move and to detect any muscle defects. For example, if the anal canal (which includes the internal and external anal sphincters) has been damaged so that it is not a complete circle, that defect (called a "guttering defect") can be seen during the anorectal ultrasound.

## Rectal Saline Infusion Test

This test measures the reservoir capacity of the rectum. It is not used very often. In the test, a measured amount of fluid is run through an enema tip into the rectum until the fluid overcomes the resistance of the sphincters. The volume of water is noted when leaks first occur. This volume is compared against a known norm, to determine whether the patient's rectum and sphincter muscles are performing as they should.

By now you probably have a good idea of what's causing your problem. If you want to know more about this, you may want to read Chapter 5 next. Or you may want to skip ahead to Chapter 6, on treatment, and then come back to Chapter 5 some other time.

# CHAPTER FIVE

# Understanding the Cause of Your Problem

*Neurological Causes* · *Muscular Causes* ·
*Anatomical Causes* · *The Special Case of Double
Incontinence*

When things are working as they should, we can retain the contents of our bowels until it is convenient to go to the bathroom. Fecal continence is preserved when the mechanical and functional factors of continence work together properly. As we'll see in this chapter, however, fecal continence can be jeopardized by any injury, disorder, or disease that interferes with the normal functioning of the factors that maintain continence.

Some people have trouble with incontinence because their sensory nerves are impaired. They may not receive their body's message that the rectum is full, or they may not receive the message until it's too late. For other people, it's the motor nerves (the nerves that send "action" messages from the brain or the spine to the muscles) or the muscles themselves that are affected more than anything else. These people have difficulty squeezing the sphincters tightly enough to retain fecal material. Sometimes nerves and muscles are both affected, and sometimes there's an anatomical problem, such as an inelastic rectum or a scarred anus, that affects function. In this chapter we'll look at the neurological, muscular, and anatomical causes of incontinence.*

Before going any further, it's important to mention that there are two conditions which are sometimes mistaken for fecal incontinence but which are not true fecal incontinence. Your physician can distinguish true incontinence from these other conditions by talking to you and examining you, and by performing diagnostic tests.

In the first of these conditions, people find that they're leaking material other than stool from the rectum, or that they're leaking stool from an opening other than the rectum. This condition is called *pseudoincontinence*. The most common causes of pseudoincontinence are hemorrhoids, sexually transmitted diseases, local anal disease, fistulas, and poor hygiene. Psuedoincontinence can be distinguished from true incontinence by the physical examination; during the physical examination, too, the cause of the problem often can be detected.

---

*Fecal impaction and loss of mobility (ambulation) are considered separately, in Chapter 7, since it's primarily elderly people and children who have impactions, and since loss of mobility is a problem that affects mostly elderly people.

Indifference, or not caring about the world around one, is another cause of fecal incontinence. A person who has Alzheimer's disease or who is mentally deficient or psychotic may not have the motivation needed to control the bowels. Fecal incontinence caused by true indifference to its social consequences requires a totally different kind of treatment that is not addressed in this book.

With pseudoincontinence, people sometimes think they're leaking stool into their underclothes when what they're seeing is actually blood or mucus. One reason people who find blood in their underwear mistake it for stool is that when blood dries, it turns brown. Another reason for the confusion is that people don't expect to find blood in their underwear, and they may automatically assume that any material in the back part of the underclothes must be stool. A doctor will be able to tell from examining the person's underwear and the perianal area that the person is leaking blood or mucus, and not stool. What's causing the blood or mucus may be clear from the physical examination; if not, the doctor may perform some tests to complete the diagnosis. In any case, the doctor will treat the cause of the problem.

A common cause of bleeding from the rectum is hemorrhoids. A hemorrhoid consists of swollen tissue that is full of dilated veins that may tear and bleed, especially when under pressure—when the person strains to have a bowel movement, for example. Pus or mucus may leak from the rectum when there's infection of any kind in the anorectal area, whether it's caused by a sexually transmitted disease, local anal disease, poor hygiene, or trauma or injury that has become infected. The passage of mucus that is slightly stained with stool is one of the first signs of a rectal prolapse, which must be treated by a doctor (see below). Fistulas are tracks (like tunnels) that may provide an artificial opening from the rectum to the skin near the anus, bypassing the anus. When stool is escaping from an opening other than the anus, the person has no control over the passage of this stool.

The second condition that must be differentiated from true fecal incontinence is frequent and urgent bowel movements. People who have a rectal prolapse, inflammatory bowel disease, or irritable bowel syndrome, for example, may feel as if they constantly need to go to the bathroom but may pass only a small amount of stool once they get there (this condition is called *tenesmus*). These people may be able to hold the stool until they are in the bathroom but may need to stay near a bathroom because they feel like they have to go all the time. Again, a physician can differentiate between this condition and true fecal incontinence.

## Neurological Causes

As we have seen, interference with the flow of messages through the nervous system can lead to incontinence. This may happen because the "sampling reflex" is not received by the brain or because the anorectal muscles don't receive the brain's message telling them how to respond to the sphincter's signal—or the muscles can't respond properly to the message. When a person's spinal cord or the nerves that come out of the spinal cord are partially damaged, for example, the flow of messages may be interrupted. Everything else in the person's digestive system may remain normal, but the person's ability to maintain continence may be compromised. He or she can stand up and get around, and the abdominal muscles are tight, and the gut is functioning reasonably well, so food is moving through the system normally, but the sphincters are not functioning sufficiently well to keep waste material back. The damage to the spinal cord or the nerves (sensory or motor) coming out of the spinal cord interferes with the normal functioning of the sphincters.

The spinal cord and its nerves can be damaged in any one of a number of ways. Tumors can cut the spinal cord or press against the nerves that come out of the spinal cord, for example, or disk disease can cause a disk to slip and damage part of the spinal cord—or a disk may be pressing up against the nerves of the spinal cord. Bony spurs from arthritis can damage the spinal cord or its nerves, as can neuromuscular disorders such as multiple sclerosis and muscular dystrophy. The spinal cord can be damaged from a lack of oxygen supply (called *ischemia*), resulting from plaques or blood clots in the arteries. Finally, an accident (such as a diving accident) can bruise, slice, or otherwise damage part of the spinal cord or the nerves that come out of the spinal cord.

The nerves controlling fecal continence can be damaged in other ways. A person who has diabetes may develop a *diabetic neuropathy,* for example; this is degeneration that affects portions of the spinal cord and its nerves and can lead to incontinence. Diabetes also may affect the involuntary nervous system to the gut, which can lead to diarrhea, especially at night. For someone who has a prolapse (see below, under "Anatomical Causes") the pudendal nerve may be stretched, resulting in injury to the nerve, which is called *pudendal neuropathy*. A pudendal neuropathy impairs the function of that nerve. Since the pudendal nerve is the major nerve that supplies the external sphincter, a pudendal neuropathy can lead to poor nerve control of the sphincter.

Someone who has a guttering defect (or keyhole deformity) also may lack full nerve control of the sphincters, because the same abscess that destroys the sphincter can also destroy nerves (see below, under "Anatomical Causes"). The physician must determine whether keyhole deformity is associated with nerve damage, because it would do no good to put a sphincter back together surgically if there weren't any nerves there to serve the sphincter.

Strokes and head injury do to the brain what these other things do to the spine. Injury to the central nervous system caused by strokes, diving accidents, and brain tumors can affect the nervous system and a person's ability to control the external sphincter. Neuromuscular disorders such as muscular dystrophy and multiple sclerosis, and also collagen disease, can affect the nervous system in a way that interferes with the factors that preserve continence.

Someone who has partial damage to the spine or the spinal nerves can be incontinent, because the gut is still functioning. The pressures from above that move fecal material through may overcome the sphincter control, which has been weakened by the neurological damage. The situation is different for someone with a spinal cord injury that causes total paralysis. Even though they have no external sphincter response (because the external sphincter is a spinal reflex, and their spinal cord has been severed), people with paraplegia are usually not incontinent. One reason for this is that their internal sphincter is still intact. This is because smooth muscle has a life of its own, has its own *intrinsic* nerves in the wall of the muscle. Its intrinsic nervous system is intact, even when the spinal cord is severed.

The extrinsic nerves that come into the intestines *modify*, or modulate, the activity in the intestines. Because of this, the activity slows down sometimes and speeds up sometimes, depending on the state of the body (whether you've just eaten, for example) and depending on the needs of the body. Without these extrinsic nerves, the peristaltic action of the intestine would just continue on without changing, and as soon as we ate, the food would come right through us.

There are spinal reflexes that can still occur even when the spine has been cut completely. Any reflexes that start out low and go down the spine will continue. But anything that requires a reflex to go up to the brain and come back down will not continue. Unlike the internal sphincter, the external sphincter must receive messages from the spinal cord in order to open.

As we have seen, defecation is a voluntary act. In order to defecate, we have to use our abdominal muscles in performing the Valsalva maneuver (straining to evacuate). People with paraplegia aren't able to do this. Because their gut is also paralyzed, they don't have propulsive forces, either. Nor can they voluntarily open their external sphincter. For these reasons, people who are paralyzed have to have an enema in order to have a bowel movement. The enema creates distention from within, and this distention causes the colon automatically to contract and push things out.

A final neurological cause of fecal incontinence is hardening of the arteries. Someone who has coronary artery disease may also have a narrowing of the arteries in the rectal area. Because the arteries are narrow, the blood supply to the area is decreased, so that it doesn't receive sufficient oxygen. Just as a heart attack can damage heart tissue and produce scarring, lack of oxygen—ischemia—in the rectal area can damage that area and produce scarring that interferes with function.

## Muscular Causes

To preserve continence, the muscles in the pelvic floor must be healthy. A healthy muscle is properly innervated—it efficiently and faithfully receives and sends messages via the nervous system—and it is intact and strong. A muscle that has been damaged may not be able to respond to messages sent by the motor nerves, or it may be weakened so that its response is not adequate to accomplish what must be done.

Muscles in the anorectal area—including the puborectalis muscle and the internal and external sphincters—can be damaged by injury or disease, or by inflammation that results from injury or disease. If the damage to the anorectal muscles is severe enough, the muscles may become incompetent—they may not be able to do what they are supposed to do. If the nerves to the muscles are damaged, then the messages of the nervous system may not be able to get to and from the muscles. When the motor nerves going to a muscle are severed, the muscle weakens and shrivels from disuse.

The anorectal muscles are perhaps damaged more often by surgical injury than by anything else. Operations like hemorrhoidectomy (removal of hemorrhoids) and fistula operations or fissurectomy are performed to correct anatomical defects that are interfering with function (see below). These are delicate operations that involve cutting into the tissue, and muscle and nerves in the area may accidentally be damaged. Industrial accidents, car accidents, and birth trauma can also injure muscles in the anorectal area.

A woman's anal muscles can be injured by a tear during childbirth if an episiotomy is not performed or if delivery is precipitous or difficult. In this case a delivery tear may go as far as the sphincter and rip the sphincter apart, causing damage that may result in incontinence, which may not begin until twenty or thirty years after the injury. It's worth noting that the woman may not remember that she had a particularly difficult time, or she may not even have been told about it. In any case, the combination of the injury to the sphincters and the tendency of muscles to become more lax, or loose, as we age can create continence problems later on.

Any injury can be complicated by infection. If infection follows injury to the anorectal muscles, the inflammation that goes along with infection may destroy the muscles even more than the original injury did. Inflammation may be caused by a bacterial or nonbacterial infection. The signs of inflammation are swelling, redness, heat, and pus. If the inflammation is in or near the sphincters it can destroy them, or it can produce a hardened scar, called an inflammatory stricture, involving the sphincters.

Inflamed tissues heal by scarring. When a scar is formed, the surrounding tissues contract, or tighten up, in the healing process. If the scar becomes hardened, then the tissues are no longer pliable or flexible. When an inflammatory stricture forms near or in the sphincter, then the sphincter becomes fixed, or hard. It can neither relax nor contract: it's frozen in a locked-open position. If the sphincter can't open widely, this sometimes interferes with evacuation. But the sphincter can't close completely anymore, either, and that leads to incontinence. With an inflammatory stricture, the sphincter becomes like a purse string that can't get any tighter than it is, and so can't close the opening.

An inflammatory stricture can occur anywhere that scarring takes place. It can occur in the intestines, for example, after the intestines have been infected, or inflamed, for any reason. If you visualize the intestines as a cylinder, then when a stricture forms, at one point in the cylinder, it gets narrower in its circumference and tightens up so that the hole (the *lumen*) itself is not its normal width, but may be one-half or one-tenth as wide as it should be. In some inflammatory disorders the lumen can narrow down to where it's pinhole-sized or even totally closed. When it gets tight enough, a stricture in the intestines produces blockages, or obstruction, but it only causes incontinence if it results in a *partial* blockage; in that case, fecal material is held up and then suddenly released and the person is unable to hold the material back. (An intestinal blockage may have to be treated surgically.)

*Inflammatory bowel disease* is the broad term used to describe inflammation of the intestines for which the cause is unknown. There are two major types of inflammatory bowel disease: Crohn's disease, which can affect both the small bowel and the large bowel, and ulcerative colitis, which only affects the large bowel. Crohn's disease is more likely to cause fistulas and abscesses in the area of the anus, and it can lead to inflammation and narrowing of the rectum. An abscess is an infection that appears as a boil, or a pocket of pus. Abscesses are caused by inflammatory bowel disease, but they also occur as a result of infection. Like any infection, an abscess can damage tissues or nerves.

One of the common symptoms of ulcerative colitis is *tenesmus,* described earlier in this chapter. Tenesmus is the feeling of a constant sense of urgency when little stool is present and little can be evacuated. It comes about because the inflammation in the rectum causes spasm that makes the person feel like there's a constant need to go, when there's actually only a small amount of stool there.

Crohn's disease usually does not affect the rectum, and the only symptom the person has is diarrhea—but even diarrhea alone, if it is severe enough, can interfere with continence. People with ulcerative colitis have frequent and bloody diarrhea. Both Crohn's disease and ulcerative colitis can affect the sphincters and also can produce propulsive, urgent diarrhea. This combination of incompetent sphincters and propulsive diarrhea almost invariably results in fecal incontinence.

When someone has inflammation of the rectum for any reason, they are said to have *proctitis.* Proctitis has many causes. One kind of proctitis, called radiation proctitis, can come from exposure to radiation. If the uterus or the nodes around the uterus or the prostate is irradiated with x-rays to treat cancer, radiation proctitis can result. In the past, when women got radium implants as part of the treatment for cervical cancer, the radiation sometimes extended to the rectum and produced inflammation there. Radiation proctitis used to occur more often than it does today, when health care professionals know how to use radiation more safely. One important thing to know about radiation proctitis, though, is that even ten or fifteen years after the radiation is stopped, the inflammation progresses as if the person were still receiving radiation.

Collagen vascular diseases can also cause inflammation that may damage the muscles or nerves or may cause strictures. There are three major collagen vascular diseases, all of them uncommon. One of them, scleroderma, affects smooth muscle, so it impairs the intestines and the internal sphincter. Lupus erythematosus also predominantly affects smooth muscle. Polymyositis, however, results in inflammation of skeletal muscle, so it affects the external sphincter and the muscles of the pelvic floor.

Myasthenia gravis is a disease characterized by weakness or fatigue in the skeletal muscles, especially after prolonged or repetitive activity. At the end of the day the person's eyelids may begin to droop, for example, because he or she has been opening and closing the eyes (blinking) all day long. This same kind of weakness similarly may affect the external sphincter and the muscles of the pelvic floor.

Two other things that can affect the muscles of the anorectal area are hyperthyroidism and aging. People with an overactive thyroid (an endocrine or hormone disorder called *hyperthyroidism*) may have muscle weakness. When the muscle weakness is severe, they may have trouble getting up from a squatting position or climbing stairs, for example. Because this condition weakens the skeletal muscles, it can weaken the external sphincter and cause incontinence.

In elderly people, incontinence can result from muscles and tissues becoming weak and lax. As we age, muscles and other tissues lose their elasticity, and they lose their strength. In addition, the nerves degenerate: as we age, we lose nerve cells throughout our body. This is why older people's reflexes aren't as good as younger people's. An older person loses muscle strength and muscle mass and reflexes in all the muscles—in the gut and the anorectal area as well as in the arms and legs. Also, people are more likely as they get older to develop diseases that can affect nerves and muscles—diseases such as diabetes, scleroderma, and multiple sclerosis. So on top of the natural effects of aging there is the tendency to get diseases that can affect continence. (See Chapter 7 for more information about incontinence among the elderly population.)

## Anatomical Causes

In addition to the nerves and muscles that control the rectum and sphincters, continence depends on the rectum and sphincters being anatomically normal. If they are structurally abnormal, or if they are functioning abnormally—or not at all—then fecal incontinence can result. The primary anatomical causes of incontinence are inelastic colon, a scarred sphincter, keyhole deformity, and rectal prolapse.*

The rectum and the colon provide a reservoir function, and anything that impairs that reservoir function can lead to incontinence. A colon that is fixed and narrow, for example, can no

---

*Congenital anatomical causes of incontinence are discussed in Chapter 7.

longer be a good reservoir. This condition, called an inelastic colon, happens when there is generalized inflammation throughout the rectum. (This is different from an inflammatory stricture, which is a narrowing of the colon in one specific area.) An inelastic colon isn't elastic and adaptive, so it can't accommodate much volume, and stool gets pushed through. Ulcerative colitis is an inflammation of the rectum and colon which impairs the visco-elastic properties of the colon so that the colon can't effectively dilate. Since the colon becomes small and rigid, it can't contain even normal volumes of stool, much less the diarrhea that people with colitis have. In this case, the loss of that reservoir function can lead to an overwhelming of the defense mechanisms for holding the stool back.

The external sphincter must be able to close up, to hold back waste material, until we are ready to defecate, so any anatomical impairment of the anus can result in incontinence. If the external anal sphincter is damaged, the anus may have what is called a *keyhole deformity*. Instead of an ellipse, the anus has the appearance of a keyhole. This keyhole deformity is like a crevice or gutter that permits waste material to leak out. This is a structural problem that often requires surgical repair.

As discussed above, the most common causes of direct injury to the external sphincter are surgery such as hemorrhoidectomy and fistula operations (especially repeated operations), industrial accidents, car accidents, and birth trauma. These injuries as well as infection and abscesses can produce a deformity in the anus. A keyhole deformity is usually discovered in the physical examination, during the digital examination (rectal examination with the finger).

A fissure, which is an open, cracklike sore in the anus, can impair function of the external sphincter. A fissure can be caused by diarrhea or constipation or by injury. Fissures can also be caused by ulcerative colitis (inflammation involving the rectum and colon) or by ulcerative proctitis (inflammation involving only the rectum). An external fistula is an open track that connects the intestines with a hole that empties onto the skin near the anus. Stool can leak onto the skin by traveling from the intestines through the fistula track to its opening on the skin. When a fistula is caused by infection, the fistula must be treated before it does damage to muscle and nerves. When a fistula results from inflammatory bowel disease, it is more difficult to treat.

Another anatomical defect is a rectal prolapse, which affects both nerves and muscles. Prolapse is caused by loose tissue, just as hernias are caused by loose muscles. Like hernias, prolapse can run in families. A prolapse begins with weak, or loose, muscles in the pelvic floor. When the pelvic floor muscles become weak, the external sphincter must work alone, and more strenuously, to maintain continence. The other thing that happens when the pelvic floor muscles are weak, though, is that the anorectal angle straightens up and is no longer held up at 90 degrees, and so the colon is almost continuously in a position of defecation. The tissues lining the colon are continually subjected to the pushes and pulls of abdominal pressure and gravity. This causes the tissue lining the intestines to slide down and turn inside out (like folding up socks or stockings). This is what's called a *prolapse*. At first the prolapse is not visible, because it is internal, but it can eventually protrude from the rectum, and it is sometimes mistaken for hemorrhoids (or piles).

As the lining of the colon is dragged down, it fills up the colon and makes the person feel as if there's a need to go to the bathroom. Once the lining distends the rectum, the internal sphincter and external sphincter relax, sensing that there's a need to evacuate. The person may strain and strain to move what he or she thinks is stool, and this straining makes the prolapse worse.

As the tissues slide, they tug on the pudendal nerve, the nerve that goes from the spinal cord to the external sphincter and helps to preserve continence. Branches of the pudendal nerve supply both the external sphincter and the puborectalis muscle, and these muscles act in unison: when one relaxes, the other relaxes; when one tightens, the other tightens. When we try to defecate, the external sphincter relaxes and the puborectalis relaxes, and by relaxing, they both open up. As the prolapse tugs and stretches that pudendal nerve, it produces a pudendal neuropathy (a damaged pudendal nerve), which impairs the function of the sphincters. The bigger the prolapse gets, the more stretched the pudendal nerve becomes, and the more damage is done. Eighty percent of people with a rectal prolapse are incontinent to some degree.

The medical history can give evidence of a prolapse, such as when a person reports leakage of stool-stained mucus from the rectum. Or if the person reports that there has been tissue protruding out the rectum, an external prolapse is suspected. An internal prolapse can be discovered through defecography.

## *The Special Case of Double Incontinence*

Many people are incontinent for both stool and urine. Having either one of these conditions is embarrassing and upsetting, but having both of them can be so difficult to manage that the person may withdraw from society and stay home all the time. Or the person may live in a constant state of anxiety, worrying that an accident will occur and will be noticed by others.

The reason so many people have double incontinence (or combined incontinence, as it is also called) is that the digestive tract and the urinary tract are closely connected, and anything that affects one of them can affect the other. First of all, the urinary tract and the digestive tract have the same embryonic origins—they start out as a single structure. Even after the digestive tract and the urinary tract separate, however, they share common nerves. Many people have both fecal and urinary incontinence because they have a disorder that affects the nerves in both tracts or because they have a disorder that affects the smooth or striped muscles needed to maintain continence for both stool and urine.

The urinary tract (also called the genitourinary tract) and the intestinal tract start out in the fetus as one single structure called the *anal tubercle*. As the fetus develops, the anal tubercle separates into two: one part, the forward tubercle, migrates forward and becomes the sphincter for the urinary tract, while the other one remains behind and becomes the sphincters for the digestive tract. The pudendal nerve brings the nerves down to these two tubercles, and then it branches. The forward branches go to the urinary tract, and the posterior branches go to the intestinal tract. The pudendal nerve is like the trunk of a tree sprouting branches of nerves out to these structures.

Because of the way they form in the fetus, then, the urinary tract and the digestive tract get their nerves from a common source, the pudendal nerve. And because they have the same innervation, anything that cuts or damages the source of their innervation at the trunk will affect both the urinary tract and the intestinal tract and may cause urinary incontinence and fecal incontinence. In other words, anything that injures the pudendal nerve high up, near the trunk, will affect all of its branches.

Any disease that affects the spinal cord or that affects nerves or muscles can affect both systems, or it can spare one of the systems. Also, the urinary and anal sphincters can be damaged by a spinal injury that affects the area above the level where the nerves leave the spine and go to the sphincters. When people are recovering from spinal cord injuries that lead to double incontinence, it's almost always the urinary system that recovers first, so it seems that the urinary system is a little more hardy than the intestinal system in this regard.

Double innervation, or the fact that the branches of the digestive and urinary systems come off of the same trunk, also makes it possible to treat both kinds of incontinence with a single technique. People who have urinary incontinence can respond to biofeedback for the anal sphincter, for example, because when they're working on the anal sphincter, they're working on the same nerve that innervates the urinary sphincter (also called the urethral sphincter). (Chapter 6 describes biofeedback training for treating incontinence.)

To find out for yourself just how closely linked these two systems are, you might try this: sometime when you're urinating, try contracting your anal sphincters. When you do, you'll find that you've cut off the flow of urine midstream, because when you contract the anal sphincters, you're also contracting the urethral sphincter. So when people learn to contract the anal sphincters, as they do with biofeedback for the anal sphincters, they learn to contract the urinary sphincter, as well. In fact, since the urinary sphincter is in the middle of the body and is not easily accessible (whereas the anal sphincter is near the opening of the body and is easily accessible), even when someone has urinary incontinence alone, it's easier to work with the anal sphincters and to expect a carry-over improvement in the urethral sphincter.

Now that you understand what's causing your incontinence, it's time to look at the options for treatment and get started in gaining control.

# CHAPTER SIX

# Overcoming Fecal Incontinence

*Behavioral Treatment • Medical Management • Surgical Treatment • When Incontinence Persists • Sexual Relations*

It goes almost without saying that a positive attitude is an essential ingredient of any medical treatment program. Luckily, for people with fecal incontinence there's a great deal to be positive about. Many, many people with fecal incontinence have overcome their problem with proper treatment. And even those who haven't entirely overcome their problem have nearly always learned to cope better, so that accidents occur less frequently or are more manageable.

Now that you understand what's causing your problem, you're ready to explore the different treatments that are available to help you take control. In this chapter, we'll describe the various medical and surgical options. You and your physician together will choose the treatment that's most appropriate for you. You'll need to keep your symptom diary up to date during treatment, so that both you and your doctor can assess the effectiveness of the treatment.

Sometimes treatment helps right away, and sometimes perseverance comes into play. If your problem doesn't immediately respond to treatment, try to keep the positive attitude that inspired you to seek help in the first place. Thinking about the gratification you'll feel when you've overcome the problem, and the marked improvement this will make in your lifestyle, will readily provide the motivation you need to try different approaches until you find the one that works for you.

## Behavioral Treatment

Behavioral treatment for fecal incontinence consists of behavior modification techniques. *Behavior modification* is a broad term that simply means "changing behavior." In this context, the behavior that we seek to change is the accidental loss of gas or stool. Two behavior modification techniques have proven highly successful in helping people change this behavior. They are *biofeedback training* and *habit training*. These are the methods used most frequently in treating fecal incontinence.

Biofeedback training can produce dramatic improvement when the cause of the problem is a lack or a loss of sphincter control or sensation—or both. On the other hand, habit training can be effective when the cause of the problem is constipation resulting in overflow incontinence. We'll discuss biofeedback training first.

The single most important factor in the successful treatment of fecal incontinence with biofeedback is that continence is a *learned automatic response*. When the internal sphincter relaxes and lets a bit of fecal material touch the nerve endings of the external sphincter, we sense the need to defecate. Our response is to close the external sphincter and make a mental note to get to a bathroom—soon, if the signal is urgent, or later, if we sense that evacuation can wait. Most people say something to themselves like "I need to go to the bathroom." Keep in mind that we *voluntarily* learn to close the external sphincter *automatically* in response to the sampling reflex of the internal sphincter. Most people first learn this automatic response through toilet training at an early age.

The point is, because we can train ourselves to close the external sphincter in response to the momentary relaxation of the internal sphincter, even some people who have never been continent for stool can learn to control their bowels through biofeedback training. For people who don't presently have control over their bowels, this is good news. It means that, with biofeedback, they may be able to learn (or relearn) this automatic response, or be successfully treated for other conditions that may be interfering with their ability to respond properly.

The purpose of biofeedback training is to train the person, first, to recognize the sensation of the momentary relaxation of the internal sphincter, and, second, to respond to that sensation by closing the external sphincter tightly enough to prevent the leakage of stool. Some people recognize the sensation of the internal sphincter but aren't able to squeeze the external sphincter tightly enough to prevent an accident; for these people, biofeedback is supplemented with pelvic floor exercises to help strengthen the response of the external sphincter and increase its competence.

In biofeedback training, what is being trained is the skeletal muscles—mainly the external sphincter but also the puborectalis muscle and the pelvic floor muscles in general. Remember that skeletal muscles are innervated by the voluntary nervous system, which means that we have voluntary control over these muscles. *We can control their function.* Biofeedback teaches the person how to control the external sphincter by measuring the action of the pelvic floor muscles and *feeding back* to the person information about how well the muscles are performing. This information is usually presented in a visual display, so the person can immediately see the effect of his or her efforts.

If you have determined that the cause of your problem is nerve impairment or unresponsive or weak muscles, then you are a good candidate for treatment with biofeedback. If you are incontinent because of a medical condition or an accidental trauma or postoperative complications—anything that interferes with the nerves or the muscles—then it's likely that biofeedback training will help you sense the signal sent by the internal sphincter, and will help you to respond appropriately to that signal. If you have both sensory and muscular impairment, treatment will start off by working to improve your ability to *sense* the internal sphincter's signal, since the muscles can only be trained to respond if there is a signal for them to respond to.

Biofeedback training can be accomplished in various ways, but most physicians use one of two biofeedback methods that have proven effective in treating incontinence. The first method is the laboratory method, which uses the same balloon device that's used in the colon motility studies described in Chapter 4. The other method is electromyographic (EMG) biofeedback. This method uses a device called a perineometer, which is also used in electromyography (another diagnostic test that is described in Chapter 4). The only discomfort that you may experience in treatment with biofeedback is from the little apparatus in the rectum. It feels like a finger examination and causes no more discomfort than a finger examination does.

You may be offered balloon biofeedback or EMG biofeedback, or both. The choice of biofeedback method you're offered may depend on what equipment the physician has and what equipment the physician is experienced with. The laboratory-administered balloon biofeedback is used first in almost all instances, however, because it is so much simpler, cheaper, and more effective.

In nearly every case, someone who is scheduled for biofeedback training has already been thoroughly examined by a physician. The physician will have taken a medical history, done a physical examination, and perhaps performed some diagnostic tests to help determine the cause of the problem. The physical examination probably included a digital (finger) examination of the rectal area. If you have *not* yet had a digital examination, however, and if you and your doctor decide to treat your problem with balloon biofeedback or EMG biofeedback, then you must have a digital examination before biofeedback training begins. The reason for this is that biofeedback training, as noted above, involves the insertion of a device—either a balloon device or an EMG probe—into the rectum. This apparatus measures and feeds back information about how the muscles are performing. Before putting such an object into your rectum, your physician needs to make sure there are no obstructions or strictures in the anus which might be damaged by the device. If the doctor feels an obstruction or a stricture during the digital examination, he or she will not attempt to insert the biofeedback apparatus.

Laboratory biofeedback, as we've said, uses a specially constructed balloon device to measure internal pressures. To begin the session, you will lie on your back or on your side. You can be dressed from the waist up, and you'll be covered by a sheet from the waist down. Once you are situated comfortably, a device with three small balloons will be inserted into your rectum: one balloon is positioned within the rectum, one in the internal sphincter, and one in the external sphincter. Each of the balloons is attached to a pressure transducer that sends a measurement of the balloons' pressure to each of three recording pens on a polygraph machine. One pen records the pressure within the rectum, one the pressure within the internal sphincter, and one the pressure in the external sphincter. The head of the bed will be elevated so you can see the tracings of the recording pens on the graph paper.

Once the balloons are in place, the physician or the technician will ask you to contract your external sphincter. He or she will measure the strength of the sphincter by recording how high the tracing from that pen goes. The physician will then tell you how much higher you need to make the tracing rise in order to be certain that the response of your sphincter is strong enough to prevent leakage. The bio*feedback* occurs when you

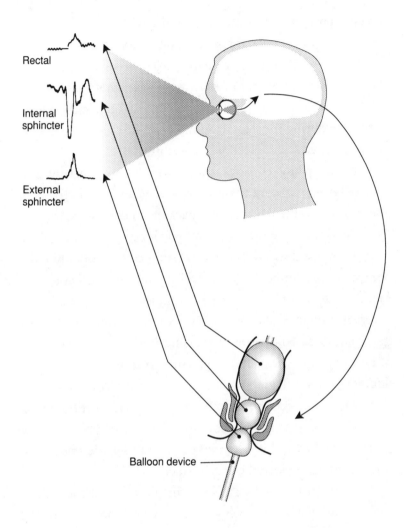

Rectal

Internal
sphincter

External
sphincter

Balloon device

*Lower left*, the balloon device used in biofeedback training. Distention of the rectum normally causes reflex relaxation of the internal sphincter and contraction of the external sphincter. During biofeedback training, the person observes the tracings of the recording pens (*upper left*) to see how well his or her external sphincter is responding when the internal sphincter relaxes.

observe the recording: you can see the tracing going up in response to your effort, and you can see how much higher the tracing needs to go.

Treatment for incontinence that relates to anal sphincter control is not just a matter of strengthening the sphincter, however. The sphincter has to be tightened at just the right *time*. If it tightens too early or too late, and is not tightened when the internal sphincter is relaxing, then you will lose small amounts of stool. To teach you to coordinate the responses of the internal and external anal sphincters, the physician or technician will artificially cause your internal sphincter to relax by pumping some air into the rectal balloon. When this air distends, or stretches, your rectum, your internal sphincter will automatically relax.

The normal response of the external sphincter is to contract in response to the relaxation of the internal sphincter, but in many people with incontinence, this response is either missing or impaired. Thus, during the biofeedback training session, the physician or technician will teach you how to contract the external sphincter exactly in unison with the relaxation of the internal sphincter. What makes biofeedback so very effective here is that the tracings show the person exactly when the internal sphincter is relaxing, and therefore the person can learn to time the contraction of the external sphincter with the relaxation of the internal sphincter.

If you have sensory impairment, the rectal balloon may need to be distended at much higher than normal levels before you can sense the need to contract the external sphincter. In the course of the session, however, the volume of rectal disten-

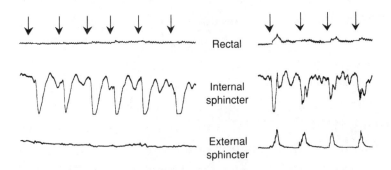

Polygraph tracings from a biofeedback session. *Left,* the tracings before train-ing show that the person's external sphincter is not responding to the mes-sage of rectal distention, even though the internal sphincter relaxes normally. *Right,* after training, the external sphincter reflex is present. It contracts nor-mally when the rectum is distended. Modified from B. T. Engel, P. Nikoomanesh, and M. M. Schuster, "Operant Conditioning of Rectosphinc-teric Responses in the Treatment of Fecal Incontinence," *New England Jour-nal of Medicine* 290 (1974): 646.

tion will gradually be reduced, until you are able to contract the external sphincter at small amounts. The biofeedback will help you to make a connection between a specific sensation in the body and the movement of the pen indicating the relax-ation of the internal sphincter. If you can squeeze only weakly at first, the amplitude of the recording pens can be adjusted so that your squeezes will register. After you have gained some sphincter strength, the amplitude will be adjusted downward, so the tracings continue to record your responses accurately.

Once you have learned to respond while watching the trac-ing pens, the head of the bed will be adjusted so that you can no longer see the pens. When the training continues, you will be asked to contract the external sphincter in response only to what you're feeling. The visual clues will be taken away from you. Your physician will continue to observe the polygraph tracings, to see how well you respond to the distention of the rectal balloon while you're relying solely on your sensation.

The contractions you will learn during biofeedback training are short-term contractions to the count of five or ten, which are followed by a rapid relaxation and another squeeze. A constant squeeze only fatigues the sphincter, and then it won't squeeze anymore, so a constant squeeze is to be avoided. Squeezing to the count of five or ten and then immediately relaxing and immediately contracting again can be done repetitively all day long—although a biofeedback session typically doesn't last even half an hour. In fact, most people learn the technique in only one 20-minute session, although sometimes several sessions are needed to strengthen the external sphincter contractions, and sometimes the training needs to be reinforced about six to eight weeks later.

As you can see, when biofeedback works, it's really dramatic, because it only requires about 20 minutes of training. When the person has learned to detect and respond appropriately to small volumes of rectal distention, the training is considered successful.

After the task has been learned in the laboratory, it's important to practice it at home. The following instructions may be helpful.

*Biofeedback instructions.* For two weeks following the biofeedback session in the laboratory, it's important for you to concentrate on your internal sensations and to squeeze the sphincter to the count of three (1, 2, 3) every time you sense anything that feels remotely like the balloon being distended, or like gas, liquids, or solid material coming down into the rectum. Make the squeeze the moment you begin to suspect that you feel something. *Don't* wait until you're sure that you feel something. That may be too late. Keep doing the squeeze-relax, squeeze-relax (holding the squeeze to the count of three) until you reach the bathroom. Stop squeezing and evacuate whatever material is present.

After two weeks you should respond the same way to any similar feelings that you sense, but you will not need to be as preoccupied with the internal sensations as you were during the first two weeks.

*Sphincter exercise instructions.* The sphincter exercises are performed exactly as you have done with the biofeedback training, except that you will not be responding to any internal sensations. You will just be doing the squeeze exercises. Squeeze the sphincter to the count of three (1, 2, 3), then relax, then squeeze again.

Do the exercises five times a day, gradually building up to a minimum of 20 squeezes at each of these five sessions. That means 20 squeezes five times a day, or a minimum of 100 squeezes a day. If you can do more, that's better. Start off by doing a few squeezes five times a day; stop when you feel slightly tired. Gradually build up the number of squeezes until you are doing the minimum of 20 squeezes five times a day. Continue these exercises for at least a year.*

Even when biofeedback training does not allow someone to overcome the problem completely, the training can bring about

*From the Division of Digestive Diseases, the Johns Hopkins Bayview Medical Center, Baltimore, Maryland 21224.

a noticeable improvement. Nancy J. Norton, who founded the International Foundation for Bowel Dysfunction to help people like herself who have fecal incontinence, relates how biofeedback training helped her:

I began biofeedback therapy, neuromuscular reeducation, with hope of gaining more physical control over the mechanisms of continence. Biofeedback therapy to date has proven to be very successful for many people. In my case the injury that I had has prevented me from having a great deal of success with the physical control of maintaining continence. Yet, I found biofeedback therapy to be very helpful to me. For the first time since I became incontinent, I felt that I was doing something that was helping me to take back control. This was a breakthrough.

Even though I could not make my anatomy work properly I learned to pay attention to my body's signals and to the cues that are all part of the mechanisms of continence. Prior to this therapy I experienced a great deal of pain due to constant spasms of the pelvic floor muscles. I was not able to relax them; I was keeping the muscles tight all the time for fear of losing stool. After learning, through biofeedback, how to relax the muscles, much of my pain subsided. Biofeedback therapy was a very positive experience for me.

As noted earlier, double incontinence (being incontinent for both stool and urine) is a common problem. People who have this problem may in fact benefit in both ways from biofeedback training of the anal sphincter. That is, their urinary incontinence and fecal incontinence may both improve with such training. The reason for this is that the sphincter at the end of the bladder and the sphincter at the end of the rectum come from the same embryological tubercle and are therefore both served by the same nerve, the pudendal nerve. When you train the external sphincter, you are also training the urinary sphincter. Even people who are only incontinent for urine sometimes train the urinary sphincter by training the anal sphincter with biofeedback, since it's such an effective method of treatment. And Kegel exercises, which are used to treat urinary incontinence, actually involve tightening the pelvic floor muscles, including the anal sphincters. (For more about double incontinence, see Chapter 5.)

Some people with urinary or fecal incontinence may be able to achieve the results of biofeedback training without formal training. If you have good sensation, you might try the squeeze exercises (to a count of three, five, or even ten, with a momentary relaxation between counts) and see whether that helps (consult the instructions on page 84). If you don't have complete success on your own, you may be encouraged to arrange for a session of laboratory training, which may be just what you need to overcome your problem entirely.

The second kind of biofeedback training for incontinence, electromyographic biofeedback, is sometimes offered instead of the balloon technique or as a backup treatment for people who don't achieve complete success with laboratory biofeedback. Some people just need some additional help—they may not yet be able to sense whether they're contracting properly, for example. And some people use this kind of biofeedback as a way of reinforcing what they've learned in the laboratory. EMG biofeedback may be used at home by people who need to strengthen their sphincter muscles and who can do the exercises more effectively when they have a visual display to provide feedback.

Electromyographic feedback is sometimes called machine-assisted biofeedback because it uses an instrument, or ma-

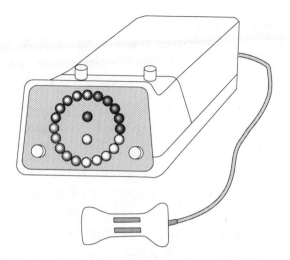

The perineometer. Colored lights are arranged in a circle on the face of the receiver. The anal plug carries signals from the muscles to the receiver.

chine, called a perineometer to provide feedback about sphincter function. The first session of EMG biofeedback training is usually done in the physician's office or a specialty clinic. To get started, the doctor or technician will insert an anal plug or probe into your rectum. This plug is a sensor that picks up the electrical signals that the muscles put out (called *electromyographic signals*). The signals are then displayed on a receiver with a circle of lights that represents the external sphincter. During training you may be fully clothed and seated comfortably in a chair.

By observing the pattern of lights on the perineometer, you can see how effectively you are contracting the external sphincter. If only one-quarter of the ring of lights comes on, for example, you'll find out immediately that the squeeze was not very effective. The amplitude of the signal can be adjusted by turning knobs on the receiver; this is useful if you have a limited capacity to squeeze at first, since unless the amplitude is adjusted, your response may not register at all. As you gain sphincter strength, the amplitude will be adjusted, so that the feedback always provides an accurate representation of your muscle function.

After learning how to use the perineometer, you can take a machine home, by either renting one or buying one. Many physicians and hospitals rent the units to patients, but if your doctor doesn't do this, you can purchase a unit or rent one directly from PerryMeter Systems, using a credit card. (Call 1-800-537-3779 for details, or write PerryMeter Systems at Biotechnologies, Inc., 6320 Bordeaux Avenue, Dallas, Texas 75209.) The cost of renting a unit may be reimbursed by Medicare or by your private insurance carrier. The perineometer can only be obtained by prescription.

Sometimes people ask about the anal plugs or probes used in hospitals or outpatient settings. These are reusable sensors that are disinfected to prevent the spread of infectious diseases such as herpes and HIV infection. If you would prefer, you can ask your doctor to order you a single-user perineometer sensor for about $150. Single-user sensors are used by one patient only and are not shared by anyone else in the hospital or by any other patients.

We turn now to *habit training,* the other form of behavior modification that is commonly used to treat fecal incontinence. As noted above, habit training is the first treatment to try if you've determined that constipation is causing you to lose control of your bowels. If you are chronically constipated, you may build up a mass of stool that becomes more difficult to pass the longer it stays in your rectum. That mass of stool may eventually cause your sphincters to relax, and when this happens, any liquid stool that enters the rectum can seep around the mass of stool and leak out of the sphincters. Because the stool that comes out is liquid, you may think you're having diarrhea, but you're really constipated. That's why this seepage is called "paradoxical diarrhea." (If left untreated, a fecal mass can become impacted and can create a condition called a *megarectum* or *megacolon*. The condition, which occurs most often in children and elderly people, is discussed in Chapter 7. Habit training for children is also described in that chapter.)

Habit training is designed to help you avoid becoming constipated in the first place. Although habit training is usually very successful for children, adults are not as flexible and malleable as children, and therefore it's harder for adults to be trained. That is, an adult's colon is used to functioning a certain way, and it may take longer to retrain it to function properly. With proper instruction, adults often can successfully train themselves, however. (Some mentally disabled adults need to work with a nurse or technician.)

Before habit training is begun, the rectum must be empty. If you have been constipated for a long time, you may need to give yourself one or more enemas to clear out stool that has built up (for directions on taking an enema, see the next section, on medical management). If the stool is impacted, you may have to see a doctor or nurse, who can remove the impaction with a finger.

Proper bowel habits depend a great deal on proper diet and exercise. Before you begin habit training, make certain you are drinking lots of water—at least eight eight-ounce glasses of *water* daily (coffee, tea, and soft drinks don't count)—and eating lots of fruits and vegetables (except bananas, which are constipating), bran, whole grain breads, and cereals. If your stool is hard and dry, you can also take a stool softener such as Metamucil, Citrucel, or Konsyl, but if you find that your stool is big and bulky, these products may make it more difficult for you to evacuate your bowels. Exercise stimulates bowel activity, so you need to try to get proper exercise.

The principle at work in habit training is pretty simple: it's that the body can be trained to react in a specific way to a regularly provided stimulus. You might think of habit training as classical conditioning, a phenomenon demonstrated by the scientist Ivan Pavlov, who trained his dogs to salivate to the sound of a bell. Another example would be the person who drinks coffee every morning to stimulate a bowel movement. That person's body learns to expect a morning dose of caffeine and may have trouble adjusting to any change in routine.

In the same way, we can train our body to get in the habit of defecating on a regular schedule. If your body expects that you will have a bowel movement regularly in response to a meal, it will gradually be trained to defecate at that time. In fact, if you're unable to sit on the toilet at your regular time, your body may let you know about the missed routine by not being able to defecate at a later time. Your body likes routine. That's

why this method of treating incontinence is called habit training—with the emphasis on *habit*.

Once your rectum is empty and you've established healthy
diet and exercise habits, you can follow the four steps below to
retrain your colon to empty regularly.

1. Sit on the toilet right after breakfast *every day*. You may
need to wake up an hour earlier than usual, so you won't have
to rush (hurrying might make you too tense to have a bowel
movement). If you can't manage a morning bowel routine,
then sit on the toilet right after *dinner* every day. By sitting on
the toilet after a meal, you're taking advantage of the fact that
food tends to stimulate bowel activity. Since your goal is to
have a regular bowel movement, it's important *not to skip a
single day,* and not to switch back and forth between breakfast
time and dinnertime. Choose one time of day or the other, and
stick with it.

2. Sit on the toilet until you have a bowel movement or
until 10 minutes have gone by, whichever happens first.

3. If you have a bowel movement, or if you had a bowel
movement the previous day, go ahead and get up after 10 minutes and resume your normal activities. If you haven't had a
bowel movement for two days, give yourself an enema or suppository after you've spent 10 minutes on the toilet the second
day.

4. Repeat steps 1, 2, and 3 until you've trained yourself to
have a regular bowel movement. You should soon be having a
bowel movement daily, or every other day, at the same time of
day. After a month or so, if you continue to need an enema
with any frequency, it would be a good idea to check with your

doctor to find out if there's something else you might do in the way of diet or exercise to stimulate your bowels.

## Medical Management

Medical management of fecal incontinence, as the name implies, involves *managing,* or controlling, your bowels so that you have bowel movements only when and where you want to. With medical management your problem is not "cured," but it is controlled sufficiently so that it no longer is a problem, or so the problem is minimized. Medical management of fecal incontinence is similar to medical management of hay fever, to use one example. If you take medication for hay fever, *you still have hay fever,* but you don't have any hay fever symptoms. If you were to stop taking your medication, however, your runny eyes and scratchy throat would return. You still have hay fever. But you are managing your hay fever medically.

The medical management of fecal incontinence is generally accomplished in one of three ways. As with behavioral treatment, you and your doctor need to choose the method of medical management that's most likely to be effective for you.

One approach to the medical management of incontinence is especially helpful for people who have trouble controlling their bowels because they have diarrhea or, more often, a combination of diarrhea and some sphincter weakness. A combination of intestinal rushes, or urgent diarrhea, and a muscular or nerve problem in the sphincters may make it necessary to control both factors. Medical management of diarrhea is sometimes combined with biofeedback to strengthen the sphincters to achieve the best result.

If you have incontinence because you have frequent urges, or rushes, especially of liquid stool, you can try using an antidiarrheal agent to suppress bowel movements. Some minor problems can be overcome by a change in diet: many people find that eating bananas, rice, and potatoes (without butter, margarine, or sauces) is enough to bind them up. For others, taking a medication may provide the answer. Lomotil, paregoric, or deodorized tincture of opium are three such medications that are available with a doctor's prescription. Another one, Immodium, may be purchased without a prescription, "over the counter."

These medications may make you a little drowsy, but most people get over that. They are sometimes constipating, and some people who take these medications reach the stage where they have difficulty having a bowel movement. The correct dosage is the dosage that controls the diarrheal rushes without constipating you. Determining the correct dosage is a trial-and-error process. Eventually you'll be able to estimate the amount that is necessary, based on your experience. Your doctor can help, too.

Some people have trouble finding the proper dosage, and some people would just rather not take medications continuously. If you would prefer, it's okay to take the medication only before you go to a social event, where you're afraid you may have an accident in public. The medication will bind you up so you can be more confident that you won't have an unexpected strong urge to defecate while you're out in public.

Controlling your bowels by controlling the aggressive forces of diarrhea may drastically reduce the number of accidents you have. This approach may even help you to overcome the problem entirely.

A second approach to medical management may be most effective for people who have accidents primarily because of a muscle or nerve impairment and who have not achieved total control with biofeedback. If biofeedback wasn't completely successful for you, you may want to manage your problem by cleaning yourself out with an enema or suppository periodically, and especially before you do anything that you know is likely to make you have an accident.

For example, one young man, a weight lifter who is partially paralyzed as a result of an industrial accident, was losing stool every time he lifted weights. That's because lifting weights is like performing a Valsalva maneuver—it increases the pressure in the abdomen. In the case of this young man, lifting weights created enough pressure to overcome his weakened sphincters. He has learned to manage this problem by cleaning himself out with an enema before doing any weight lifting.

One problem with this method of bowel management is that many people who are incontinent can't retain an enema or a suppository. Because the anal sphincter isn't strong enough to retain the water (in the enema) or the suppository, it comes back out. If this happens to you, you may need to try other methods of retaining the water or the suppository long enough for them to work. One possibility is a colostomy irrigation kit, which has a cone instead of an enema tip. This cone can be pushed up against the anus, and it will prevent water from coming back. Or you can insert an enema tip or suppository and then squeeze your buttocks together with your hands until you've retained the water (or the suppository) long enough for an effective response.

An enema makes a person have a bowel movement because the water from the enema creates pressure in the colon which moves the stool out. It also makes the stool more liquid. A suppository works by softening the stool and stimulating the bowel.

Here's how to give yourself an enema or a suppository. (If you choose to use a suppository, we recommend that you use glycerin suppositories unless something stronger is needed, in which case a Dulcolax suppository is recommended.) Before you begin, put a rug in the bathroom and lie down on it, on your left side. Insert the enema tip (or the cone or the suppository), and hold the enema bag a foot or so above your body. (Once the enema bag is empty, you can remove the tip and the bag. If the bag is not completely empty, lower it or clamp the tubing before removing the tip.) Lie there as long as you can—until you feel that you can't control it anymore—and then get up on the toilet and evacuate your bowels. You'll need to use a trial-and-error approach to determine how high to raise the enema bag. Keep in mind that the higher you hold the bag, the faster the water goes in. Raise the bag or lower it, depending on how much pressure you want.

The third method of medically managing incontinence involves the use of a device called an anal stimulator. Again, this management technique is most effective for people with impairment of the anal muscles or nerves.

Anal stimulators were used more frequently in the past, before the success of biofeedback, which has proven to be much faster and more effective. If you are still having problems after biofeedback training, you might try using an anal stimulator. In truth, though, only a very few people who don't respond to biofeedback will respond to this device. If the sphincter is capable of functioning, biofeedback makes it function. When biofeedback doesn't work, it's because there are no nerve connections or because there's not much sphincter left. The anal stimulator can work without nerves, but if there is a large scar and if there is no muscle left, it might not work.

The stimulator consists of a small power pack and an anal probe to stimulate the sphincter muscles. To use the device, you keep the probe in all day, or all night, and walk around with the power pack in your pocket. The power pack powers the electrical stimulator in the anal probe which provides a continuous stimulus, just as a pacemaker provides a continuous electrical stimulus to the heart. By stimulating the sphincter muscle to contract, this device keeps the muscle toned up and can increase its strength over time. It takes three to four months for the device to work. At present its drawbacks include skin irritation and the mild discomfort of walking around all day with a plug in. With improvement in the future, however, devices such as this might be more effective.

## Surgical Treatment

Medical treatment should almost always be tried before resorting to surgery. When nothing else works or when there is a structural defect, like a gap in the sphincter, then surgery may be helpful. Unfortunately, surgery for fecal incontinence hasn't proven terribly successful, for reasons we'll discuss below. Before you have anal surgery, then, it's important to prepare yourself psychologically for a partial success or even a failure.

If you have a gap in your sphincter (from an obstetrical injury, for example), then the anal circle is incomplete. Sometimes biofeedback can help you overcome this defect, especially if there isn't a wide gap and the ends of the muscle are very close together. The muscle can sometimes compensate and overcome that gap by strengthening itself. If it doesn't, or if the gap creates a guttering or crevice defect, then you will have leakage of gas or stool.

If the defect is severe, or if you can't live with the symptoms, you may need surgery to repair the defect. Unfortunately, every time surgery is performed it produces a scar, and a scar produces a gap, which is another defect. Because there's a scar instead of a functional muscle, and because a scar will get smaller in time (it will shrink as it heals), the scar may create a keyhole deformity (see Chapter 5). Then you may need plastic surgery to repair that defect. But even plastic surgery doesn't always work.

Beyond surgical repair of anal defects, there are several other kinds of surgery used in the treatment of fecal incontinence. The simplest approach, called *anal encirclement,* is one of the least effective. Anal encirclement involves implanting a device called a *Thiersch ring* into the anal opening. In this operation the surgeon takes a wire or a plastic suture and makes a ring down at the anus and closes the anus like a purse string. The reason this ring doesn't work very well is that it is nonfunctioning. You can't tighten it when you want to tighten it or release it when you want to evacuate. It is static and unchanging—it stays there as it is.

After anal encirclement surgery, the person will need to use enemas in order to have a bowel movement. The enema is needed to create enough forcefulness, and make the stool liquid enough, so that the stool can flow through the partially closed ring. Not surprisingly, since it can't be tightened, the ring can leak. This makes it a pretty ineffective treatment for fecal incontinence, one that is seldom used anymore.

Another approach to anal surgery is a muscle transplant, which involves taking a small muscle and making a new sphincter out of it. This approach has not been terribly successful, either. In recent years, however, British surgeons have been trying a new method of muscle transplant, in which they isolate a small sliver of muscle from one of the leg muscles and then stimulate it with an electrical current to make it contract, or squeeze down. After they've conditioned the muscle to act in this way, they implant it in the place in the circle where the sphincter is weak. This surgical treatment for incontinence is most successful if the person uses a continuous stimulator (as described in the preceding section) to keep the muscle tight. When the person wants to have a bowel movement, he or she cuts off the stimulator and the muscle relaxes.

When fecal incontinence is caused by problems with the sphincter, but sphincter problems are caused by other problems—for example, a prolapse—then surgery would be performed to repair the problem that's interfering with the function of the sphincters.

Colostomy surgery is sometimes performed when fecal incontinence is severe and doesn't respond to medical treatment and can't be effectively managed otherwise. We discuss colostomy surgery, among other approaches, in the next section.

## When Incontinence Persists

For some people, fecal incontinence continues to be a problem even after medical treatment or surgery, although treatment may decrease the severity or frequency of accidents. As we noted earlier, medical treatment or surgery isn't successful for everyone, and it isn't *for* everyone. Sometimes the medical cause of incontinence makes it unlikely that any of the methods described so far in this chapter will be helpful. Although new treatments for fecal incontinence are being investigated all the time, many people must come to terms with the fact that incontinence is a problem they're going to have to reckon with. By learning to *minimize the impact* of accidents, many people with this problem lead active, normal lives.

People who successfully minimize the impact of fecal incontinence use a combination of products and techniques to contain, mask, and camouflage accidents. There's no question that finding the right combination may be a challenge, especially for an active person who is regularly away from home or who exercises or takes part in other physical activities. As with many things in life, however, it's essential to *be prepared*. Take the time, make the effort, and find out what works for you. Then you can leave your home in confidence, knowing that you have a way to take care of things should an accident occur.

Before describing some of the products and techniques that are available to help people with an ongoing problem, it's worth repeating something we said in Chapter 1. That is that many people with fecal incontinence deny that they have a problem, even to themselves. Denying that the problem exists is a natural and understandable reaction, and denial is made easier if accidents occur only occasionally. But people who deny that they have a problem are not likely to be prepared to deal with an accident when it occurs. People who admit that they have a problem and prepare themselves to handle an accident if one should occur usually feel better for having taken control of the situation.

Family members, friends, spouses, parents, and others need to understand that it takes some people longer than others to get to the point where they're ready to admit that they have a problem, and that no one can decide for someone else where that point is. No one can force anyone else to admit there's a problem if the person is not ready to do so. Gentle suggestions or offers of help are usually accepted better than demands, however. You may want to leave information about products or support groups lying around where the person is likely to see it. Or you may decide that it's best to back off and wait until the person is ready.

If you are a person who loses control of your bowels, whether occasionally or frequently, whether by losing a small amount of stool or a large amount, there are many products available that may help you manage these accidents. And there are many organizations available to help, too. The people who answer the telephone at these organizations often understand from personal experience what it's like to have this problem. If you call one of these organizations, you'll probably find that the people on the other end of the telephone listen sympathetically and offer good advice.

The "Additional Resources" section at the end of this book lists several organizations that provide services to people with fecal incontinence. One of these organizations, called HIP, Inc., publishes a resource guide (called "Resource Guide of Continence Products and Services") which describes a variety of devices that may be useful to people with urinary or fecal incontinence. The guide describes disposable, reusable, and skin care products, as well as other devices, and tells you how to obtain them. (You can obtain a copy of the guide by contacting HIP, Inc., at P.O. Box 544, Union, South Carolina 29379.)

Among the many disposable products available are absorbent underwear (brand names include Attends and Depends) as well as underpads to use on a bed (such as Chux, which are manufactured by Johnson and Johnson). Reusable products include diapers, reusable briefs, and reusable underpads. Most people use a combination of these products to help them contain accidents. Some people find that there's no ready-made product that's quite right for them, however. These people have taken control of the problem by improvising: they use sanitary napkins, for example, or compressed cotton plugs obtained from a dental supply store. Different people have different needs—again, it may take some experimenting before you find a combination that works for you.

If you're worried about having an accident while you're away from home, then it's a good idea to wear a protective undergarment of some kind when you go out. It's also a good idea to take along the supplies you'll need for cleaning up if an accident occurs, as well as a change of clothing and of whatever undergarments you use. Nancy J. Norton, the founder of the International Foundation for Bowel Dysfunction, describes how she leaves home fully prepared for an accident:

I carry a large handbag (a briefcase or sports bag would also work). Inside are several changes of protective undergarments, underwear, cleansing cloths, water bottle, disposable plastic bags to hold soiled articles, tissue, medicated skin cream, a moisture barrier cream, and cleansing cream. I will often carry a briefcase or another bag with a change of clothes. I wear a lot of black clothing because it's easier to change pants or a skirt discreetly if it is the same color. I have been able to find what works for me and all the things that I need to have "just in case." At times I feel encumbered by all the paraphernalia, but I also feel more confident that I can manage my incontinence.

In addition to wearing protective undergarments and carrying the supplies you need to clean up after an accident, you might want to take dietary precautions against gas and odor. We know that certain foods create gas and tend to make the stools have a strong odor. By avoiding these foods, you can decrease the chances that a small accident will be noticed. Even a large accident is less embarrassing if there is no odor. You might want to avoid the following foods, especially if you find that they give you a problem (adapted from "Diet and the Ostomate," by Michael Gold, M.D., in *Proceedings of the Conference on Rehabilitation,* edited by Marvin M. Schuster [American Cancer Society, Maryland Division, September 1979]):

| *Vegetables* | *Protein* | *Other* |
|---|---|---|
| broccoli | eggs | fried foods |
| Brussels sprouts | chicken | vitamins |
| cabbage | fish | gum |
| turnips | beans | sodas |
| cauliflower | | mushrooms |
| sauerkraut | | beer |
| cucumbers | | mustard |
| radishes | | pickles |
| asparagus | | |
| onions | | |
| peppers | | |

One way to render fecal material less odorous is to take an internal deodorant containing chlorophyllin copper. Derifil, Nullo, Whoo-Noz, Nilodar, and Odoban are examples of these pills, which are taken by mouth. Ask your pharmacist about these products. If you take any of these internal deodorants, you should be aware that they may turn your stool and urine green. Some people worry about the long-term effects of taking these products, too, and you may want to use them only when you are going to be out in public. Don't take more than the recommended dosage.

Finally, skin care is very important for anyone with fecal incontinence, because the skin around the anus and bottom will come into contact with fecal material during an accident, as will the hands during cleanup. And fecal material can be irritating to the skin—especially liquid material, because digestive enzymes are still present and active in material that has traveled through the digestive system quickly. The external deodorants that are used to eliminate or mask the odor of feces can also irritate the skin, and some cleansers can, too, especially those containing soap, which is sometimes difficult to rinse off completely.

Using a medicated cleanser is the first step in cleanup. Choose a cleanser that is soapless and nonirritating. If you find a cleanser that contains moisturizers, deodorizers, and a fragrance *and that doesn't irritate your skin,* then go ahead and use it if you want to. But watch for any signs that these ingredients are breaking down your skin. If this happens, or if you develop an allergy to the product you're using, then switch to another product right away.

Using a moisture barrier to protect and soothe the skin in the perianal area is very important. Keeping the area dry will discourage the growth of bacteria and fungi, both of which can cause severe irritation or infection. There are a variety of products to choose from, in liquid or cream form, all of them specially designed for use by incontinent people. Powders that are designed to absorb dampness are also helpful, but, again, choose one that doesn't contain any ingredients that you know you are allergic to.

If you develop a severe skin rash or irritation, or if you have any indication that the skin is infected (warmth, swelling, discoloration, or pain or severe itching), get in touch with your doctor. Depending upon how familiar your doctor is with your problem, and how well your doctor knows you, he or she may prescribe something for you over the phone. But the doctor may want to see you, to determine the exact nature of the problem and to determine whether there's any sign of maceration, a process where the skin begins to break down.

If your problem does not respond to any of the treatments for fecal incontinence described in this chapter, and if you find that anticipating and cleaning up accidents is consuming all of your time and energy, then you may be a candidate for colostomy surgery. Colostomy surgery is the only completely successful surgical treatment for fecal incontinence, and it is only recommended for people who have a serious loss of sphincter control. If because of an automobile or other accident a person's nerves are cut completely and don't regrow, for example, or the muscles are destroyed and cannot be replaced, then medical treatment and medical management are unlikely to help. If you have fecal incontinence because of a problem such as this, you may want to consider colostomy surgery.

In colostomy surgery, the surgeon brings the large intestine out onto the abdomen through an opening in the abdomen. A pouch is attached to this opening to collect stool. A colostomy can eliminate incontinence because there's no longer any need to worry about soiling, because feces are collected in the pouch.

One thing you should know about a colostomy is that you have to have a certain amount of dexterity to manage the appliance. People with arthritis or people who don't have the mental capacity to handle things just can't manage the colostomy. You'll also need to have a certain amount of equipment on hand, and you'll need to learn how to change the pouch and clean the area. Ostomy care is very important for your health.

Keeping the area around the opening free of infection and fungal growth, for example, requires special attention. Surgeons who perform ostomy surgery often have someone on their staff who can provide specific instructions for using the special products that have been developed to care for this area. An ostomy support group can also be very helpful for those who are newly learning to care for an ostomy.

For some people colostomy is the only answer, and they find that it gives them freedom to socialize and travel and do all kinds of things they weren't able to do when they were constantly worried about accidents. But many people have trouble accepting a colostomy, and there's no doubt that it requires a psychological adjustment. Before you have colostomy surgery, ask your doctor to explain exactly what's involved, and to answer any questions you have. Read about colostomy surgery and colostomy care, and contact an ostomy support group (see "Additional Resources," at the end of this book). The people who belong to these groups can tell you what it's like to have an ostomy, and they can help you in other ways, too.

## Sexual Relations

It seems appropriate to close this chapter with a brief discussion of sexual relations. The reason is that this is an area of life that is often overlooked when discussing a problem such as fecal incontinence. Sexual expression is a pleasurable part of most people's lives, however, and it is only natural for people with a problem like fecal incontinence to worry about how the problem will affect their interest in and ability to take part in sexual activities. They may worry even more about how the problem will affect their partner's interest in the sexual side of the relationship. Or how and when to tell a prospective partner about the problem, and how the person will react.

Studies have shown that men who have had colostomy surgery most often worry about how the surgery will affect their ability to perform, and women worry more about whether their partner will still accept them and desire them. But it's reasonable to think that *all* men and women, whether they have medical problems or not, worry about *all* of these things at one time or another. Studies have also shown that the people who adjust best to problems like this are the people who were pretty well adjusted before the physical problem happened.

In other words, if you functioned well sexually before you became incontinent, and if your partner found you desirable before you became incontinent, then the chances are good that you and your partner will find a way to overcome the obstacle of fecal incontinence. You may work around the problem by cleaning yourself out before getting intimate, or by taking a constipating medication. If this isn't possible, then the only thing to do is to deal honestly with an understanding partner who can put you at ease and who can cope if you should happen to have an accident. This will take some getting used to, and some practice, but with time, it's possible for your sexual life to return to normal.

Adjusting one's sexual life to accommodate fecal incontinence is difficult. But for some people, a problem like fecal incontinence shows them just how much they care about each other. The problem doesn't "belong" to one person or the other but to both of them, and they work together to overcome it. For other people, though, the picture is different. Some partnerships can't survive the stress of fecal incontinence—or kidney disease or multiple sclerosis or any other problem, for that matter. The fact is, if the relationship has some serious weaknesses to begin with, then any kind of stress can bring it to the breaking point. And if the relationship is strong, then the relationship is likely to survive this problem and many others much more serious. The emotional well-being and the degree of attachment of the people involved have a lot to do with that.

# CHAPTER SEVEN

# Special Considerations for Children and Elderly People

*Incontinence in the Very Young · Incontinence in Elderly People · Fecal Impaction and Megacolon · Bowel Training for Children*

This chapter will focus on the special issues having to do with incontinence in children and elderly people. Children have this problem half again as often as the population at large, and fecal incontinence is much more common among elderly people than among younger adults. The problem also can be somewhat different for elderly people than it is for other adults. Both children and elderly people with fecal incontinence have special needs.

In this chapter we'll look at the most common causes of fecal incontinence among these age groups, paying special attention to fecal impaction and megacolon, a frequent cause of fecal incontinence among both children and elderly people.

We'll consider how children and older people with this problem can be helped, and we'll describe a bowel training program that has been successful for many children.

## Incontinence in the Very Young

A child who is older than four years of age and who does not have control over his or her bowels can be considered to be incontinent. For such a child, the problem of incontinence is very real indeed. The child may shy away from other children, for example, or be reluctant to go to school because he or she is afraid that the other children will tease, or the teacher will scold, if he or she has an accident. If the child has been teased in the past or has been reprimanded by an unthinking adult, the child's reluctance to take part in activities may turn into real resistance. If this problem goes on for very long, it may affect the child's personality and social development. It will certainly affect the child's self-esteem.

Whether the child's family has handled the problem with understanding or not, the child's own embarrassment may lead him or her to take extreme measures to keep the problem a secret, even from the family. A child who is embarrassed or afraid of discovery may leave soiled underwear where the child hopes it won't be found: in the woods on the way home from school, for example, or in the department store bathroom. It's not unusual for such a child to hide soiled underclothes in dresser drawers, closets, or shoeboxes. A parent who finds soiled underwear hidden away needs to find a way to help the child without adding to the child's sense of shame and embarrassment.

When a child is incontinent, the rest of the family usually suffers, too: they probably feel a variety of emotions, including sympathy and concern for the child as well as embarrassment, guilt, and anger. They suffer because of the inconvenience, because they're embarrassed over what other people might think, because they're worried about what's causing the problem, and because they're anxious and frustrated over their inability to help the child overcome the problem. These are legitimate causes for concern.

Some parents also worry that fecal incontinence is a sign that their child is emotionally disturbed, but this is usually not true. This concern is probably left over from the days when fecal incontinence was thought to result from emotional problems. A child who was incontinent was thought to be psychologically or emotionally disturbed, and the child's parents were often blamed for improperly parenting the child. It was thought that the parents' mistakes in raising the child were causing the child's emotional problems, and that the child was "acting out" these emotional problems by refusing to use the toilet properly.

After studying many children with fecal incontinence over many years, however, doctors now think that emotional disturbance accounts for fecal incontinence in only a minority of children who have this problem. This means that while incontinence may *cause* emotional problems (as discussed above), it's less likely that emotional problems are the cause of the incontinence. This is important news for parents, who formerly may have gone to great lengths to keep the child's problem a secret from neighbors, friends, or even the child's physician because they were worried that they would be blamed for the problem. Parents who understand that the child's incontinence is probably not the result of an emotional problem—and, even more important, that the problem may be easily corrected—are more likely to seek help for the child. However, whenever emotional problems do play a role, it is important to address them as early as possible, before they become deeply rooted.

Most children who are incontinent are now considered to be incontinent because of a *physical problem* that is interfering with normal fecal continence. It is only when the child shows clear signs of having an emotional disorder and there are no signs of an organic cause that an emotional disorder may be considered the primary cause of incontinence. And this must always be differentiated from an emotional *response* to incontinence. In the following paragraphs we'll discuss the physical causes of incontinence in children.

First, a word about the word *encopresis,* which is the formal term for fecal incontinence. This word was once more widely used than it is today, and there is still controversy over its proper use. Many parents and grandparents probably associate the word with fecal incontinence resulting from an emotional disturbance or improper toilet training. In that sense the word has sometimes had a negative connotation. Today, some experts suggest that this term be used *only* when someone has fecal incontinence with no detectable organic cause. Other experts don't use the word *encopresis* at all, and instead use the term *fecal incontinence* to describe the problem, regardless of its cause. In this book we have chosen the latter usage.

The underlying problem that causes incontinence in children most often is constipation. As we shall see, constipation can lead to incontinence because it creates a *mechanical* problem (a partial blockage). *Physical* problems that are present from birth (called congenital abnormalities) also cause incontinence, either directly or indirectly, through constipation, in a small percentage of children.

To say that constipation is the most frequent mechanical cause of incontinence in children probably seems paradoxical. Constipation, after all, means unnaturally *retaining* stool. But in children and in adults, constipation can cause what is called *overflow incontinence*.

Here's what happens: If the child has an abnormally functioning bowel (a sluggish colon, say) from birth, the child will not evacuate his or her bowels as often as needed. Or the child may go off to school for the first time and may decide that he or she doesn't want to use the school bathroom, or doesn't want to spend as much time in the bathroom as is needed to produce a bowel movement. The bathrooms in many schools don't provide much privacy, or they're dirty or smelly; sometimes, too, children tease each other in the bathroom, and many children will keep away from the bathroom to avoid being teased. Another cause of constipation is painful fissures, which may make a child avoid having a bowel movement. Medicines such as the decongestants used for sniffles and colds can cause constipation, too.

Whatever the cause, as the days go by and the child doesn't

have a bowel movement, fecal material will build up. The longer it stays in the colon the harder it will get, too, as more and more of its liquid content is absorbed. Then the child, who already has difficulty moving his or her bowels, will find that passing this large, hard stool is very difficult and perhaps even painful. If the stool is very large, it may tear the anus and create a fissure (a little split in the anus), making defecation even more painful for the child from then on. The child then avoids moving the bowels, producing more constipation and more pain, and this creates a vicious cycle.

Under these circumstances the child will try just about anything to avoid having a bowel movement, and the problem will get worse. When the child retains the stool and has large volumes of stool in the rectum that he or she has been holding back for various reasons, the stool may become impacted, which means that the child will not be able to move the stool out without assistance. If the impaction builds up and becomes large, eventually liquid stool will flow around the solid stool; this is called a *paradoxical diarrhea*, or overflow incontinence. (Fecal impaction can eventually also lead to a condition called a *megacolon*. Fecal impaction and megacolon and their treatment are discussed later in this chapter.)

Parents very often bring a child to the pediatrician because the child is soiling his underclothes with liquid stool. They think the child has diarrhea, but frequently the child's real problem is constipation, which is causing a paradoxical diarrhea or overflow incontinence. The treatment for overflow incontinence, as we shall see below, is very different from the treatment for diarrhea. When you treat the real cause of the incontinence—the constipation—you also get rid of the "diarrhea" and incontinence. More and more pediatricians are beginning to recognize paradoxical diarrhea as overflow incontinence, but parents, too, need to be aware that seepage of liquid stool does not always mean that the child has diarrhea.

Some congenital abnormalities cause incontinence. One of the more common of these is spina bifida. This condition results when the spinal cord in the embryo doesn't close over. Because the spinal cord remains open and fails to develop completely, some of the nerves don't develop appropriately and don't reach the areas they are supposed to reach. During normal fetal development the nerves come from the spine and migrate down to the muscles. If that migration is arrested, and the nerves don't reach the muscles, then the muscles aren't innervated, and they may not be able to function as they need to in order to preserve continence. Children with myelomeningocele, the most severe form of spina bifida, often have fecal impaction and megacolon. Studies have shown that many incontinent patients with spina bifida can learn to have normal bowel movements and avoid accidental soiling when they are given proper biofeedback training. Some children with this condition are helped by being given enemas or suppositories on a regular basis. This keeps their rectum relatively empty so that the internal anal sphincter alone can prevent incontinence.

As we saw in Chapter 5, spinal cord tumors can destroy the nerves by putting pressure on the spinal cord or occupying space where the spinal nerves ought to be. Children are sometimes born with a tumor on the spinal cord, and this can make them incontinent.

One of the problems that can exist from birth is a rare congenital anorectal anomaly called an *imperforate anus*. When a child is born with an imperforate anus, the lower end of the gastrointestinal tract doesn't develop properly, and there's no opening to the outside. Rather than opening to the anus, the colon ends in a blind sack. In all human embryos, the gastrointestinal tract starts off as a closed, solid cord, and as it grows it begins to hollow out. If it doesn't become hollow, then it doesn't allow an opening. Also, the intestinal tract develops in two directions in the embryo: it comes down from above and up from below. It's like building a tunnel beginning at two ends and in different directions, and the tunnel has to meet in the middle.

If this development is stopped early in the development of the fetus, the two ends don't meet. If this happens later in fetal development, the two ends are joined but there's still a slight film closure over the anus. If that's the problem, a simple surgical cut creates the opening. If the two ends get very close together but something stops the development before the two ends meet, then there's a septum up higher; in this case, the surgeon takes those two openings and joins them by sewing them together.

How does an imperforate anus cause incontinence? First, when there's arrested development of the kind that causes an imperforate anus, often the nerves have not developed properly, either, and they haven't come down and contacted the muscles properly. Second, the sphincter muscles may not be there, or they may be very flimsy and underdeveloped. Third, surgical repair of an imperforate anus is very delicate, and it's impossible for the surgeon to avoid cutting some nerves, since there are nerves all over the place. The surgeon can't cut the tissue, separate it, and then bring it back together without doing some damage to nerves. If the surgeon hits the trunk of a nerve, like the pudendal nerve, then the surgical repair of the imperforate anus can result in damage that can cause incontinence. If the surgeon hits some of the branches of the nerves, then less damage is done. If the damage is minor, the child learns on his own to compensate; if not, the child may need biofeedback training to help him or her recognize what the problem is and how to solve it. In surgery for severe imperforate anus, the surgeon replaces the rectum with a section of bowel, and the reservoir capacity of this section of bowel may not be nearly as good as the reservoir capacity of the rectum, so the child's ability to retain stool may be impaired.

There is some evidence that fecal incontinence is transmitted within families, so having a mother or father or siblings with the problem increases the likelihood of any individual child's being incontinent. It's not clear whether the problem is transmitted genetically or behaviorally (through social learning), though experts think that the tendency to be constipated may be inherited genetically.

Finally, some children do seem to deposit their stool in the wrong place deliberately. Even this behavior can sometimes be due to the child's fear of painful defecation, however. The child who has been successfully using the toilet for some time but then has a painful bowel movement, perhaps because of a particularly large or hard stool passed after a temporary bout of constipation, may subsequently resist using the toilet for fear of repeating the painful experience. With the intention of helping the child avoid just that, the parents may demand that the child sit on the toilet and produce a bowel movement, perhaps at a time when the child has no urgency to do so. A power struggle may ensue, with the child choosing to defecate in inappropriate places rather than give in to the parents' demands that he or she use the toilet.

Sometimes toilet training is the source of the problem. Parents may have been too strict, they may have chosen the wrong time to try toilet training, or they may have done something to cause the child to associate use of the toilet with something painful, unpleasant, or frightening. Sometimes toilet training is begun before the child is ready, and then the parents' expectations will not be met. Just as an infant six months old cannot be made to walk, no matter how much training and coaching he or she gets, a child younger than eighteen months cannot be toilet trained. Most children are past their second birthday before they are fully trained, with many children not being trained until age 3 or older.

A time of emotional upheaval in a family is not a good time to teach toilet habits, either, and events such as divorce, death, a new sibling, or a move to a new home can be expected to interfere with progress. A child who has been properly using the toilet for some time may "relapse" and begin having accidents when there's something stressful going on in the family. Some children have trouble paying attention to their body's signal, and they may find themselves too far away from a toilet when they feel the urge to defecate. Some children are afraid of the toilet, or of something they imagine dwells in the toilet, or of falling into the toilet—and they may resist toilet training for this reason.

Even when the child is physically and mentally mature enough to be trained to use the toilet, however, accidents during toilet training are not unusual. Parents who react to accidents by punishing or scolding or even spanking the child may find that the child avoids having a bowel movement because the child is afraid of the consequences if he or she doesn't make it to the toilet in time. To avoid punishment, the child may retain feces and, as a result, become constipated. In this case, when the child does finally move his or her bowels, defecation may be painful, and the cycle of retention and painful defecation begins.

A child may be thrilled to use the potty, or he or she may decide *not* to use it, as a way of keeping control over oneself, despite what the parent wants. The child may deposit stool in inappropriate places as a way of "showing" the parents that they can't control this aspect of his or her life. Soiling may be the child's way of expressing independence or getting revenge. Deliberately thwarting his or her parents' clearly expressed desire for the child to use the toilet may also be the child's way of getting attention. Children can't withhold money or otherwise punish their parents, but leaving stool in the wrong place is a pretty effective way of letting parents know that *something* is wrong.

Regardless of how a struggle over toileting develops between a child and his or her parents, depending on the child's age and temperament, as well as on the family's situation and way of handling things, such a struggle may either be easily negotiated and quickly resolved—or settle into a long-term battle in which neither side wins. Confronted with this behavior, parents would probably be well advised to consult a psychologist or psychiatrist who specializes in treating children. The solution may be as simple as delaying toilet training or waking the child up earlier in the morning so he or she has time to use the toilet at home, before going off to school. If there are emotional reasons for the child's behavior, such as when the child is having difficulty coping with a life event, then the specialist can help the child and the rest of the family understand and solve the problem.

A bowel training program for treating incontinence in children is described later in this chapter. Children above 6 years of age who are incontinent can also be trained with biofeedback techniques, described in Chapter 6.

## Incontinence in Elderly People

The older we get, the more likely we are to lose the things that are most dear to us: our spouses and friends; our financial independence; the ability to drive and otherwise get around without assistance. With age often comes illness, too, and other conditions brought about by the aging process. One condition that many elderly people develop is incontinence; in fact, elderly people are more likely than any other segment of the adult population to be incontinent for stool and urine. Some older people are able to cope emotionally with incontinence, and they cope physically by wearing adult diapers. Or they may seek medical help for the problem. However, many older persons view incontinence as one more loss, one more sign that they are losing control over their lives. Such persons may even feel as if they are regressing to infancy again. They may get depressed, and they may stay at home rather than face the possibility of having an embarrassing accident. If they have any physical illnesses or conditions, depression can make the symptoms of the illness worse.

The family of an incontinent older person may eventually decide that he or she can't live at home anymore, and they may put him or her in a nursing home. Most fecally incontinent elderly people are placed in nursing homes. In fact, incontinence is the second leading reason for putting elderly people in nursing homes. Once there, the older person may feel as if he or she has totally lost control over his or her lifestyle and has given up (or had taken away) the last vestiges of independence. This may cause an even deeper depression, and the elderly person may stop making any effort to take part in life, including making any effort to control the bladder and bowels.

The National Nursing Home Survey* found that nearly 30 percent of nursing home residents were incontinent for stool. Eighty-seven percent of these people were also incontinent for urine. Restricted mobility may be an important factor. Data from this same survey indicate that 60 percent of elderly nursing home residents who were put in restraints were fecally incontinent, and 41 percent of those in wheelchairs were fecally incontinent, whereas only 17 percent of nursing home residents who could walk with a cane or a walker had the problem.

*J. F. Van Nostrand et al., *The National Nursing Home Survey: 1977 Summary for the United States*, DHEW Publication no. PHS 79-1794 (Washington, D.C., 1979).

Social indifference or mental incompetence may also play a role, since 56 percent of residents with mental illness or dementia were fecally incontinent, while only 21 percent of those without mental difficulties had the problem. From this information it's clear that fecal incontinence is a common problem among older adults living in nursing homes, especially if they have trouble getting around or if they have any cognitive difficulties.

The most significant cause of fecal incontinence among older people is neither loss of mobility nor dementia, however. It is simply the natural effects of aging on the body. One of the natural effects of aging is weakening of muscles and tissues, which can lose their elasticity and strength and become lax. In addition, nerves degenerate as we age. Neurologists have figured out how many nerve cells we lose in our brain every day—but the fact is that we lose nerve cells throughout our *entire* body. This explains why an elderly person's reflexes aren't as quick as a younger person's. Also, the longer we live, the more likely we are, too, to develop any one of a number of diseases, like diabetes, scleroderma, or multiple sclerosis, that can affect nerves and muscles and thereby cause incontinence (see Chapter 5).

As we age, we lose muscle strength and muscle mass and we lose reflexes, and these changes affect what happens in the anorectal area just like they do in any other area—the arms and legs, for instance. An older person can't lift as heavy a load or carry a heavy load as far as he or she could at a younger age, because of the loss of muscle strength and mass. Similarly, some older people can't retain gas or stool, especially liquid stool, as well or as long as they were once able to, because the muscles in the anorectal area have become lax. Also, the older person may not be able to reflexively close the external sphincter quickly enough to avoid an accident. Compared to continent elderly people, incontinent elderly people have less rectal sensation and less sphincter strength.

Impaired mobility accounts for fecal incontinence among a large proportion of older adults, and it can cause incontinence whether the person is in a nursing home or not. Someone who has had a stroke, or someone with arthritis who finds it painful to move around and therefore moves very slowly, may not be able to get to the bathroom in time to avoid an accident. And anyone who is wheelchair bound may have trouble getting to the bathroom and onto the toilet. Sometimes even good physicians fail to recognize that the cause of incontinence for these individuals is not the sphincters but the fact that they can't get to the bathroom. The more immobile the person is, the more likely it is that he or she will be incontinent.

In some nursing homes the problem of lack of mobility is compounded by the problems of nursing home care. If the person is strapped in a bed or a chair and can't get around, or the person has had a stroke or has arthritis that doesn't permit him or her to get around, simple immobility on the part of the patient prevents getting to the bathroom. If the person has repeatedly called the nurse, and the nurse repeatedly does not arrive with the bedpan in time, or in time to help the person get to the bathroom, the person will almost certainly become discouraged or angry and stop calling. Then he or she will just go ahead and "make" anyway. In nursing homes as in private homes, continence in an older person who has limited mobility depends at least in part on how nearby the bathroom facilities are and how readily available help is to get there. Family members and friends, the nursing home staff, and physicians often don't think about that, and they blame the incontinence on the person's age or state of mind. When the immediate family and other caregivers are understanding and supportive, the elderly person is more likely to recover from illnesses and is more likely to have a positive outlook that may affect his or her willingness to try to regain continence.

Another common cause of fecal incontinence in older adults is stool retention. As we have seen, very young children often retain stool, as well. While we often don't know the reason for stool retention in a child, in an elderly person stool retention is usually due either to a lifestyle that creates a condition of constipation or to lax muscles that make it difficult for the person to have a bowel movement.

When a person slows down due to age or illness, the decreased amount of physical activity can lead to stool retention, even if that person has not had a problem with constipation in the past. Physical activity helps to move things through the body; conversely, lack of physical activity slows things down. When the digestive process slows down, the stool tends to remain in the colon longer, becoming harder the longer it stays there, and more difficult to move out.

Constipation can also be caused by improper diet, and by some medications that elderly people take, such as the medications commonly prescribed for Parkinsonism. Many older people have sore gums or false teeth that don't fit properly, or they may be missing teeth. Such a person is unlikely to eat all of the foods that are necessary for a healthy diet. Some elderly people don't have enough income to buy fresh fruits and vegetables, either, or they find that preparing these foods takes too much effort. Or they live alone, or they have lost the spouse who used to do the cooking, and they just don't feel like making the effort to prepare meals. Whatever the reason, a diet that lacks fiber can cause constipation. Sometimes people self-treat their constipation by taking laxatives. Over time, using laxatives can interfere with a person's ability to defecate on his own, too. Developing bad habits of any kind can create a vicious cycle, because stool that has been retained is more difficult to move out. Many older people develop these bad habits for one reason or another.

The other reason older people are likely to retain stool is that their muscles have become weak. In order to have a bowel movement, we contract the abdominal muscles and exert pressure on the diaphragm, which descends like a piston in a cylinder and increases the pressures in the abdomen (see Chapter 2). If those pressures are increased sufficiently, both the internal and the external sphincters open up so we can defecate. Consider this, however: if the piston comes down in a tight cylinder, the pressures are increased; but if the piston comes down and the cylinder sags out, no additional pressures are created. That's what happens if the abdominal muscles are weak: they just sag, and even when the person strains to have a bowel movement, there's not enough pressure. When the muscles in the gut get weaker and the nerves get impaired, things don't move out as readily. If a person can't strain down

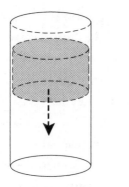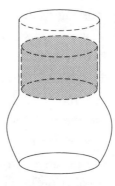

When a piston comes down into a weakened cylinder, the pressure inside the cylinder doesn't increase, because the cylinder just sags out. When the diaphragm descends into an abdomen with weakened muscles, pressure inside the abdomen doesn't increase enough to move the stool out.

properly, the person may not have enough strength in the voluntary bowel muscles surrounding the abdomen to evacuate. The muscles inside the colon also weaken as we age, and this can slow the movement of stool through the colon and contribute to constipation by allowing the stool to remain in the colon so long that it becomes dried out.

Chronic constipation may lead to fecal impaction, and this in turn can create a condition known as *megarectum* or *megacolon*. Megarectum and megacolon cause incontinence in the very old and the very young.

## Fecal Impaction and Megacolon

The most common cause of fecal incontinence in children is chronic constipation. But when it results in an impaction, chronic constipation causes problems for children and elderly people both. When a person retains a large amount of stool, it builds up into a mass that can become the size of an orange or a grapefruit, even in young children. When a person has an impaction, the physician who performs a digital (finger) examination will almost invariably find that the person's rectum is stretched and is full of stool.

As discussed above, a child may retain stool for any number of reasons. An elderly person usually retains stool because rectal tissue gets loose and muscles become lax and nerves degenerate, and the rectum becomes distended. When a child or an adult retains stool for a long time, eventually the lining of the rectum may become stretched, and this can produce a megarectum (an enlarged rectum). If the stretching extends higher than the rectum, the person develops a megacolon (an enlarged colon). It's been estimated that these conditions are responsible for fecal incontinence in a whopping 80 to 96 percent of children who are incontinent for stool.

Megarectum or megacolon causes incontinence in two ways. First, the mass of hard stool in the rectum or colon chronically inhibits the internal sphincter and, to a lesser extent, the external sphincter, so that the natural "pursestring closure" that is usually provided by the sphincters is not functioning properly. Recall that in their normal resting state, the internal and external sphincters are both closed, and that in order to have a bowel movement we need to open them by applying force downward. What happens when the rectum or colon remains full of stool for a longer than normal period is that the sphincters remain relaxed, and open, all the time. Under these conditions, liquid stool can seep around the impaction and leak out of the person's sphincters. Second, the impaction makes it difficult or impossible for the person to be able to sense that small amounts of new stool are moving into the rectum. The impaction impairs the person's rectal sensitivity, so the person may not feel the urge to defecate.

In other words, when someone has an impaction in the rectum, the impaction has the same effect as straining to have a bowel movement. There's a large pressure in there, produced by this massive stool, and the massive stool expands the rectum to the extent that the rectum sends a message to relax both sphincters so that evacuation can take place. None of this is sufficient to produce evacuation of the impaction, because moving stool out requires the proper functioning of an intricately coordinated process. But it paves the way for evacuation, and as a consequence there's no obstruction down below from a tight sphincter. When new stool comes into the colon the stool is soft, because it hasn't had a chance to harden or dry out. When that new, soft stool flows around the impaction, it's able to escape from the body through the sphincters, which are relaxed in response to the "full" message from the rectum.

When this soft or liquid stool escapes, what results is a paradoxical diarrhea. As noted earlier in this chapter, many people who appear to be having diarrhea are actually having overflow incontinence, which means that a small amount of soft or liquid stool is flowing past the hard, dry stool that is being retained in the colon and rectum. The elderly person with impaction and the parents of children with impaction see this soft stool and think it's diarrhea, but it's not diarrhea, it's really constipation producing a paradoxical diarrhea.

To treat the problem, first, the impaction must be removed

(this is called *disimpaction*). Sometimes this can be accomplished with enemas, but if the impaction is very large it may have to be removed by a doctor or nurse with a finger. Once the impaction has been removed, the rectum or colon usually returns to its previous shape if the bowel is kept relatively empty through regular bowel movements. Also, when constipation is adequately treated, the overflow incontinence usually stops immediately. The second step in treating the problem, then, is to change the diet or develop toileting habits that produce regular bowel movements, to prevent the buildup of stool.

To avoid impaction, elderly people who have hard stool should add bulk to their diet with foods such as vegetables and fruits (except bananas), bran, whole grain breads, and cereals. They can also take a stool softener such as Metamucil, Citrucel, or Konsyl (there are many brands). But in elderly people who have impaction because they don't have good muscle strength and muscle movement, the impaction may be very soft, and it may be huge and bulky; these people don't *need* to add bulk to their diet, since that will only make the impaction larger. They need to improve the propulsive forces, by using enemas or stimulant laxatives. Elderly people should never take mineral oil to treat constipation, because they can aspirate it (get it into their lungs) and develop oil pneumonia.

Children don't need more bulk, either; their diet has lots of bulk. Whatever the cause of a child's constipation—a sluggish bowel or a battle over toileting or an impaction—nearly every child can overcome the problem with behavioral habit training. In fact, nearly 90 percent of children who have received this training have been helped this way. That's the subject of the next section.

## Bowel Training for Children

In children the treatment of fecal incontinence that results from constipation and megarectum is known as *behavioral habit training*, or habit training or bowel training. (For a child who has already been trained to use the toilet but who has regressed, it may be retraining.) Bowel training for children essentially means teaching the child to evacuate. The parents give the child an assist with a suppository or an enema when necessary, but the child is first given the option of having the bowel movement on his or her own, without help.

We recommend that parents consult their child's pediatrician whenever a child is having a problem with incontinence, just to be certain that there's no underlying physical problem. If the pediatrician finds that impaction and megarectum are causing the child's incontinence, the pediatrician will probably recommend bowel habit training.

It's a good idea for parents to stay in touch with the pediatrician during the training. We also recommend that parents keep a symptom diary for the child (see Chapter 3). Be sure to keep track of the number of accidents, occasions when the child stains his or her clothes, and normal bowel movements on the toilet. In this way the child, the parents, and the pediatrician can keep track of the child's progress. The pediatrician may want to make adjustments in the training program as the child's habits improve—or fail to improve.

Success takes longer in some children than in others: studies show that most children require only a few weeks of training, but some require a year or longer. If parents feel that not enough progress is being made, or that progress is being made too slowly, they need to consider whether they're being impatient. Children are quick to pick up on a parent's impatience, even when the parent thinks he or she is hiding it, and the child's sense that the parent is impatient may interfere with progress. On the other hand, if the parents have faithfully followed the program and believe that the child is not making adequate progress, they may want to express their concerns to the pediatrician. The pediatrician may consult a specialist in bowel habit training, or, if the child's case seems particularly difficult, the pediatrician may refer the parents and child to a specialist who will work intensively with them.

Some physicians recommend treating constipation and overflow incontinence in children by giving them mineral oil, but we believe that mineral oil ought to be avoided unless it's the only thing that works. Certainly other treatments, such as habit training (described below), should be tried first. The reason treatment with mineral oil is undesirable is that it creates a terrible mess. Parents are instructed to give the child enough oil to make the child literally incontinent. Mineral oil then leaks all over the clothing and furniture, and since the oil leaches the fat from the stool, and that fat is orange, what comes out is a very messy orange discharge. (As noted above, elderly people should generally avoid mineral oil because of the danger of oil pneumonia.)

Before bowel training begins, any impaction must be removed. Often this can be accomplished by giving the child laxatives or enemas (your doctor will advise you), but sometimes the doctor will need to use a finger to disimpact the child. Once the bowel is emptied, the training program keeps it empty, so the child's rectum or colon can regain its normal shape and tone. Keeping the bowel relatively empty usually puts an immediate stop to overflow incontinence, as well.

Also before bowel training begins, the parents and the child have to come to an understanding. You should tell the child what the purpose of the training is, and try to get him or her excited about the prospect. Depending on the child's age, you might say that this training is like other kinds of physical training people do to get in shape, such as aerobics or weight lifting. Describe the daily routine, and define success for the child: success is having a bowel movement on the toilet or not having an accident for an entire day. Explain what the reward will be for success, and try to minimize failures. Explain all of this in a matter-of-fact way, and then ask the child whether he or she has any questions. A written contract between parent and child may help sometimes, to make sure that everyone understands—and remembers—what behaviors will be rewarded, and how they will be rewarded.

Here's how the training works.

1. Place your child on the toilet right after breakfast *every day*. It may be necessary to wake up a school-age child an hour earlier than usual, to allow an unhurried routine. If that's not possible, then place the child on the toilet right after *dinner* every day. The reason for placing the child on the toilet after a meal is to take advantage of the fact that food tends to stimu-

late bowel activity. Since the purpose of the training is to teach the child to have a regular bowel movement, it's important not to skip a single day, and not to switch back and forth between breakfast time and dinnertime. Choose one time of day or the other, and stick with it.

2. Ask the child to sit on the toilet until the child has a bowel movement, but *no longer than 10 minutes*. If the child's feet don't touch the ground, place a footstool under the feet to make pushing easier. If the child doesn't know how to push, teach him or her how. You might blow up a balloon, and then ask the child to blow up the balloon, or blow into a party horn. If the child does this properly, she or he'll get the idea of how to bear down to have a bowel movement.

3. If the child had a bowel movement the previous day, she or he can get up after 10 minutes and resume normal activities. If the child hasn't had a bowel movement for two days, then give an enema after he or she has spent 10 minutes on the toilet the second day. You'll find directions for giving an enema to a child immediately after these training directions.

4. Have the child check her or his underpants at the same time every morning, and you check the underpants often during the day. Do this matter-of-factly, and don't embarrass the child or try to make a joke about it. If the child's underpants are clean, praise him or her and provide a treat such as a piece of candy, some small change, or a promise of time spent doing a favorite activity with a parent or a special friend.

If the child's underpants are soiled, instruct him or her to clean up by putting the bowel movement in the toilet (if it's large), washing out the soiled underwear and putting it in the clothes hamper or washing machine, and cleaning herself or himself and putting on clean clothes. If the child dawdles, give a reminder to keep going but don't nag or get angry. The child may need your help in cleaning up the first couple of times, but after that he or she should be able to clean up without your aid. Record the accident in the symptom diary.

5. If the child has a bowel movement in the toilet on her or his own, *without having an enema,* reward with praise and a treat. Some children like to be told that important people in their lives, like grandparents or even cartoon characters, will be glad to hear about their success on the toilet. You can also have a "star chart" or some other system for keeping track of successes; you can tell the child that after accumulating several "stars" or successes, he or she will earn a large reward, such as a trip to the amusement park or a trip to the store to buy a special outfit. Record the bowel movement in the symptom diary.

Studies have shown that rewards are most effective if they are given immediately, consistently, and with an explanation. Smile at your child, and say how pleased you are that he or she has had a bowel movement in the toilet, and has not had an accident. Once the child begins to make progress, you'll need to make it a little more difficult to earn the large rewards. You and the child can agree, for example, that from now on, it will take five stars in a row instead of only three to be rewarded with a game of mini golf with his father or another favorite relative, or perhaps with a friend. If the child is as pleased with his or her progress as you are (and most children are), she or he will probably accept the new challenge gladly. Remember that successful habit training takes longer for some children than for others. Improvement may be noticed almost immediately or only after several weeks or months of training.

As mentioned in step 3, you may have to give your child an enema as part of the program. Enemas work by distending the rectum and making the child feel the need to have a bowel movement; in addition, they clean out stool that has been held in the rectum. You can buy Fleet plain water enemas (with salt additives) at the drugstore, or you can use plain tap water in an enema bag. Check with your doctor about what's best for your child. Use about 1 ounce of water for every 20 pounds of the child's weight. Unless recommended by your doctor, do not use more than 4½ ounces of water. There are other products to treat constipation, but we recommend water enemas. Nevertheless, those other products are described below.

Before you give an enema to your child, be sure to explain what you will be doing and what can be expected to happen. Then have the child lie down on the left side on a towel or mat on the bathroom floor. Put Vaseline jelly on the tip of the bulb or the enema tip, and also coat the child's anus with Vaseline jelly. Help the child relax by telling him or her to take long, slow breaths.

Gently insert the bulb about one inch into the anus and slowly squeeze the water into the rectum. Do not add the water too quickly, because that can make the child uncomfortable. If an enema bag is used, it should be held about one foot above the child's body. Hold the child's buttocks together to keep the water inside the rectum until the child tells you he or she needs to have a bowel movement. The enema should take effect within 20 minutes.

Suppositories work by softening the stool and stimulating the bowel to eliminate. If you prefer to use a suppository, we recommend that you first try glycerin suppositories. If this doesn't work, you can use a Dulcolax suppository, which usually produces a bowel movement within 45 minutes. To give your child a suppository, have the child lie on the left side; remove the silver paper and insert the suppository about 2 inches into the bowel. Hold the child's buttocks together until he or she tells you he or she has to go to the bathroom. If after 20 or 30 minutes the child hasn't mentioned the need to go, you can have her or him sit on the toilet until a bowel movement is produced.

As mentioned in the previous section, children with normal eating habits and a normal diet usually do not need any additional bulk in their diets, so we recommend that you *not* give your child bulk laxatives. Unlike an enema, which produces virtually immediate results, commercial laxatives can take as long as 12 hours to work. Again, we recommend that you avoid them altogether for your child. If you like, and if your child will cooperate, you can give your child extra portions of vegetables and fruits, especially prunes (and avoiding bananas, which are constipating), as well as whole wheat cereals and brown breads. These foods help stimulate bowel activity.

Sometimes bowel habit training alone is not sufficient, and in that case biofeedback training, as described in Chapter 5, can be added to the training program with excellent results.

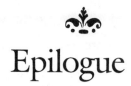

# Epilogue

*As you can see, if you have a problem with fecal incontinence, there are many things that can be done, many ways in which you can be helped. There's a total package for treatment which includes attitude, motivation, sphincter training, sphincter-strengthening exercises, medications, and, occasionally and when indicated, surgery. When treatment is not entirely successful there are products that can help you manage. Treatments and products are being improved all the time. Don't give up.*

*The basic ingredient that is required for everything is a strong positive attitude and a strong motivation to overcome the problem. When you do, there's great gratification in having overcome the problem, and a marked improvement in your lifestyle. We know one person who is putting her strong positive attitude and motivation to work for other people. This is Nancy J. Norton, the founding director of the International Foundation for Bowel Dysfunction, a nonprofit organization begun in 1991 to address the issues surrounding living with a functional bowel disorder, including incontinence. Nancy Norton wrote the Epilogue that follows.*

It's difficult to imagine the devastating impact incontinence can have on a person's life without experiencing it directly. By sharing my own experiences, as well as those of others who live with fecal incontinence on a daily basis, I hope to contribute to a better understanding of this disorder: how it can affect a person's life, and how it can be managed.

I was 35 years old when I became incontinent due to an obstetrical injury. As a new mother, I was faced with caring for my child and trying to take care of my own medical needs. During the first few months of my son's life I underwent two surgeries for repair of my anal sphincter muscle and my damaged pelvic floor. Psychologically, I was distraught. The physical pain was hideous.

As time passed with no change, I would often wake up hoping that maybe today I would be continent, that somehow the surgery had done what the doctors had hoped it would do. But as weeks and then months went by, it became clear that although my anatomy had been repaired, my continence had not been restored. I kept thinking that there had to be a solution, because I could not possibly live the rest of my life like this.

Continence is something that we take for granted, not thinking about it until something goes wrong. Yet, from the time I was a young child I knew that incontinence could affect a person's life. My mother had multiple sclerosis which caused a loss of both bladder and bowel continence. She fought hard to maintain her dignity. Twenty-five years ago, people did not talk about this subject. Unfortunately, things have not changed much. This is still a disorder that people feel they must hide from others and talk about only in whispers.

When I first became incontinent, I too spoke in whispers, weighing every word, because the topic seemed to make other people uncomfortable. Their discomfort made me anxious, and my anxiety often triggered a response in my gut that itself could lead to an episode of incontinence. It took some courage just to talk about it. To then be met with a lack of sympathy or with indifference and in some cases disgust was like being pushed back even further into myself where my words were guarded and a part of my identity was concealed. It was an uncomfortable pattern, a circular path leading nowhere. Before I would be able to begin to learn how to best cope with and manage my incontinence, I would have to break out of this pattern of retreat.

Initially I felt that there were many things I could not possibly do because I was afraid I would not have access to a bathroom. I isolated myself by staying home, where I felt more secure. To leave the house meant confronting my incontinence. By staying home I could avoid dealing with many of the issues I dreaded. An episode of incontinence would be upsetting at home but would have been devastating in a public place. I was on the road to isolation, thinking that I could build my life around staying home. I had lost my self-confidence, I had lost the image that I had of myself, and I feared that my sexuality was threatened. My life had changed in such an abrupt and unwanted way; I was unable to see the new me emerging because I was struggling so hard to hang on to my perception of the person I had been. It quickly became apparent, though, that denial was not a choice that I was going to be happy with. There were things that I needed to deal with.

Managing incontinence means confronting and dealing with issues involving uncertainty, loss, and control. Of these, uncertainty may be the most difficult. Being incontinent means forever living with uncertainty. Not knowing when or where an episode of incontinence will happen causes a great deal of stress and anxiety. In *Healing and the Mind,* Bill Moyers writes: "Uncertainty is the worst illness. The fear of the unknown can really be disabling." Incontinence may happen once a month, once a week, or several times a day. The extent of control or lack of control is different for everyone, but emotionally all people with incontinence are faced with coping with the loss of a bodily function. Bowel management for incontinent people is a 24-hour-a-day job.

Some people are able to get themselves on a fairly routine bowel program. They are able to empty their bowels on a regular basis and feel comfortable and relatively assured that their bowels are under control. There are others, like me, for whom this is not such an easy task. For people who also have irritable bowel syndrome, diarrhea, constipation, gas, and pain, and for women who experience diarrhea associated with their menstrual cycle, or for those who experience sensory loss, incontinence can seem overwhelming.

A friend once suggested that someday I'd look at incontinence as more of an inconvenience than as something that is ruling my life. The comment made me angry at the time. Incontinence is much more than an inconvenience. Yet, there was something in what my friend said. At that time I was letting the uncertainty surrounding my inability to control my bowels have control over every aspect of my life. I needed to separate the issue of uncertainty from the issue of control. *As long as I am incontinent, I will live with uncertainty, but how I manage my incontinence is something I must and can control.*

Loss is a characteristic of being incontinent. Different people feel this loss differently. Carol is a 36-year-old engineer, a professional who enjoyed her work and active life. When she became incontinent after routine rectal surgery, she described feeling overwhelmed by sadness and personal loss, including the loss of "personal, professional, and physical freedom and spontaneity."

Most people with incontinence share these feelings of loss. For me, coping with the loss meant that I had to go through a process involving several stages of emotion. It was important not to allow myself to get stuck in any one of these stages. There were stages of denial, anger, grief, and finally of gaining the ability to take back control of my life in the best way I could. Taking back control meant empowering myself, and giving myself permission to say, "There are things I can do and things I can't do, and if I can't do something I don't have to try to hide it or feel bad about it." Regaining control of my life was a gradual process.

Kathy became incontinent after having back surgery. She describes a roller coaster of initial emotions: "Fear, disbelief, shame, guilt, depression, panic, and anger took turns shattering my ego. I spent countless minutes, hours, and days trying to convince myself that this must be a flu, something I ate, my digestive system is just weak from surgery, as soon as I can walk better or am stronger this will go away, because I am *not* incontinent! Each time I soiled my clothes, bed, floor, carpet, or myself, I felt worthless, helpless, and completely devastated. I cried endlessly until I was too exhausted to stay awake, then slept fearfully thinking and trying not to think, 'What if I have another accident?' I spent hours in the bathroom hoping to avoid another accident. Incontinence consumed my time, my thoughts, my life."

With any disability, I think, the initial reaction is to focus on our own view of our personal loss. As I learned to recognize my incontinence as only one part of myself, however, it began to take its place among the many facets of who I am as a whole person. For one thing, I am a member of a family, and incontinence is something that affects the entire family. It has brought change into the lives of my husband and son as well. I have been fortunate to have a loving and supportive husband, but the effect on my relationship with my husband was manifested in many ways. Going to a park with friends, taking our son to the zoo, or going out for an evening became challenges. Discomfort, fear of an episode of incontinence, and diminished self-image interfered with the more personal and intimate parts of our relationship. I not only had to learn how to cope with all the things that were different about me but I also had to be able to express these things to my husband. He needed to understand why our everyday life was being affected and what we needed to do together to get back to a more normal life.

He was willing to work through the changes with me, but I needed to be open with him about what I was going through and what my needs were. Communicating our individual needs is important. Sometimes this is not easy to do. I sought professional guidance, and this helped me with some of the issues I was struggling with. Communicating and sharing often takes courage, especially in the confusion and chaos of adjusting to the sudden onslaught of incontinence.

Kathy: "Being incontinent means being honest with friends, family, and myself. It means accepting the fact that some people in my life will never be comfortable with my incontinence and being strong enough to realize that some relationships will come to an end because of this, but new relationships will take their place."

Living a life with incontinence means getting past the dread of being incontinent in public and understanding that nothing is as bad as the dread you impose upon yourself. It means being prepared. With preparation comes confidence, as Kathy found: "I can recall the first time I was incontinent away from home. I locked myself in a public bathroom stall with no intention of coming out. Before long I heard my husband's voice and there he was in the women's bathroom with me, quietly saying, 'It's all right, you have to come out, Kathy, you can't stay in there forever. What can I do to help you?' He went to the store and bought me new clothes so I could clean up and change for the drive home. It took me quite a while, but when I was finally ready to try leaving home again I left with clothes and supplies to handle an accident away from home."

Few people can be so candid about what fecal incontinence means to them. We all must struggle with our emotions while we manage our incontinence.

Looking back, I think what I needed most was for someone to acknowledge my loss and not just expect that it was something that could be dealt with by trying to empty my bowel in some routine manner. In trying to sort through different alternatives, I realized that I needed to set some priorities for myself. It was time to make my own decisions.

Biofeedback training and relaxation techniques, combined with emotional support from my husband and a few friends, helped me to get back into life and participate in the way I wanted to. It was not something that happened overnight. It involved a long process of self-investigation and motivation. I read the medical literature regarding my own particular injury and incontinence. I felt it was necessary to educate myself as much as possible about my particular situation. I soon realized that I wasn't the only woman who was incontinent after the delivery of a child. It became evident that there is a significant proportion of the population who are incontinent, yet there is very little information for such people.

I looked for support groups, hoping to find one that could help me. I attended meetings and sent for literature from several organizations, but I just did not fit into those groups, so I continued to search for people and look for information that I thought could offer me more insight into living with my incontinence. I suspected that if I felt the desire for information and support, others like me would be interested, as well. I felt that there needed to be an organization that could provide educational information and support for people like me. I explored the concept of forming an organization for several years before I finally formed the International Foundation for Bowel Dysfunction (IFBD). I think that I was committed to doing this long before I acknowledged it to myself, although I was not sure if I could deal with my own incontinence on a daily basis while facing the challenges that I anticipated the foundation would present. Yet, I knew there was a need, and I felt driven to try.

I recently came across this passage in "Living Your Dreams," an article in *Lotus* written by Frederic Hudson: "A dream is like a haunting refrain. You know that you have one when it won't let you go and others are attracted to it within you. You know that you have a vision when it seems already to be guiding you toward its reality and you don't have to explain it to yourself." My dream was for an organization, a voice, with the strength to speak out about the issues facing those with incontinence, to remove the stigma attached, and to educate and empower those affected.

In order for IFBD to become an effective voice, I needed support from the medical community. I am grateful that a number of physicians and therapists active in the field of functional bowel disorders agreed that this was an area that needed to be addressed and offered their support. We have since established a medical advisory board of some of the most noted authorities on bowel dysfunction. IFBD includes among its members concerned physicians, psychologists, nurses, and occupational therapists who are all contributing their time and effort so that the foundation can offer useful information to individuals with the problem and to health care providers.

The organization started with just a few very courageous people calling or writing to me. For some, it was the first time they felt they could open up and talk to someone about their experience with fecal incontinence. We have laughed and cried together and come away with a sense of comfort in knowing that we are not "the only one."

Tom, now a college student, was in a bike accident at the age of 13. After living with a colostomy for several years, he had the colostomy reversed and found that he was incontinent. Despite having an operation on his sphincters (sphincterplasty), he still experiences incontinence. After all his many struggles, he sums up his feelings regarding his incontinence this way: "Life is so full of wonderful things I hate to think of what I would be missing if I had let myself get stuck in a phase of denial or self-pity."

A lack of information, a lack of understanding, can be just as damaging as denial or self-pity. Seek information. Find understanding. Incontinence does mean making lifestyle changes and compromises. But it does not have to control you or rob you of a full life.

In my own life a twist of fate changed the course of my future. Incontinence is not something that I ever imagined I would be faced with, as a young and healthy adult. Incontinence changed my life, imposed itself upon me, and almost took control. But I fought back, and I keep fighting back. I want to live my life to the fullest. And I will continue on, all the time learning more about this unpredictable thing called incontinence, maintaining my grace and dignity along the way.

*You can contact the International Foundation for Bowel Dysfunction by writing to IFBD, P.O. Box 17864, Milwaukee, Wisconsin 53217, or by calling 414-964-1799.*

*If you have questions that relate to this book, you might take the book to your physician. He or she might be interested in seeing it.*

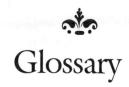

# Glossary

*Abscess:* An infection that appears as a boil or a pocket of pus.

*Anal sphincters:* The muscles in the anus. See also *External anal sphincter* and *Internal anal sphincter*.

*Anal stimulator:* A device consisting of an electrical power pack and an anal probe. It stimulates the sphincter muscles and may increase their tone and strength over time.

*Anorectal angle:* The angle between the rectum and the anus provided by the puborectalis muscle.

*Anorectal ultrasound* (also called *sonography*): A diagnostic test used to detect muscle defects. In ultrasound, sound signals are bounced off internal organs or muscles to produce an image of these organs or muscles on a television screen.

*Anoscopy:* A diagnostic test in which the physician looks at the anus through an instrument called an anoscope.

*Anus:* The final two inches of the rectum, surrounded by the internal anal sphincter and the external anal sphincter.

*Barium enema:* An x-ray study of the colon.

*Behavior modification techniques:* Methods used to teach or train people to change their behavior.

*Biofeedback training:* A behavior modification technique in which a person receives a visual or auditory signal (the "feedback") that indicates how well the person's muscles are responding to the commands of the person's nervous system. Biofeedback training for fecal incontinence is most effective when incontinence is caused by loss of sphincter control or loss of sensation.

*Bowel movement:* The act of passing feces through the anus.

*Bowels:* Another word for *intestines.*

*Colitis:* A kind of inflammatory bowel disease which affects the large bowel, or colon. One form is *ulcerative colitis.*

*Colon* (also called *large intestine* or *large bowel*): The last part of the digestive system, which absorbs liquid from feces and moves fecal material to the rectum.

*Colon motility studies* (also called *manometric tests* or *manometry*): Measurement of pressures and movements within the colon.

*Colonoscopy:* A diagnostic test in which the physician looks at the colon through a flexible instrument.

*Congenital abnormality:* A physical problem that exists at the time of birth.

*Constipation:* A condition in which the feces are hard and dry, and elimination of feces is difficult and infrequent.

*Continence:* The ability to retain feces until it is convenient to have a bowel movement.

*Crohn's disease:* A kind of inflammatory bowel disease which can affect both the small bowel and the large bowel.

*Defecate:* The act of having a bowel movement.

*Defecography* (also called *proctography*): A diagnostic test in which x-rays are taken of the muscles in the anorectal area.

*Diabetic neuropathy:* A condition in which portions of the spinal cord and its nerves have degenerated as a result of diabetes.

*Digestive system:* A system made up of organs in the body that extract liquid and nourishment from food and eliminate the waste material that's left over.

*Disimpaction:* The act of removing stool from the rectum which could not be eliminated normally. Enemas, suppositories, laxatives, and finger extraction are all means of disimpacting stool.

*Electromyographic (EMG) biofeedback* (also called *machine-assisted biofeedback*): In biofeedback training to treat fecal incontinence, this is a method that uses recordings of electrical activity from muscle contractions.

*Electromyography:* A diagnostic test used to measure the electrical activity of the muscles.

*Encopresis:* A formal term for *fecal incontinence*.

*Esophagus:* The organ connecting the throat and the stomach (also called the gullet).

*Evacuation:* Another word for *bowel movement*.

*External anal sphincter:* A voluntary muscle in the anus which contracts in response to rectal distention to prevent defecation and which relaxes to allow defecation.

*Fecal incontinence:* The accidental and involuntary loss of liquid or solid stool or gas from the anus.

*Feces:* Waste material from the intestines. Feces are composed of bacteria, undigested food, and material sloughed from the intestines.

*Fissure:* A tear or an open, cracklike sore in the anus.

*Fistula:* A track of inflammation that bores a hole through tissue.

*Flatulence:* The release of gas through the anus.

*Gas:* Material that results from swallowed air or that is created when bacteria in the colon break down waste material. Gas that is released from the rectum is called *flatulence*.

*Gastroenterologist:* A doctor who specializes in diagnosing and treating disorders of the digestive system.

*Habit training:* A behavior modification technique in which the body is trained to react in a specific way to a stimulus. Habit training for fecal incontinence is most effective when constipation is causing overflow incontinence.

*Hemorrhoid:* An enlarged vein in the lining of the anal canal.

*Hemorrhoidectomy:* Surgery for the removal of hemorrhoids.

*Hyperthyroidism:* A condition that develops when a person has an overactive thyroid.

*Impaction:* A blockage in the rectum composed of a large amount of dried stool that is difficult to evacuate. See also *Disimpaction*.

*Incontinence:* The accidental and involuntary loss of stool or urine. A person may have fecal incontinence or urinary incontinence or both (sometimes called *double incontinence*). See also *Fecal incontinence* and *Urinary incontinence*.

*Inflammation:* Swelling, redness, and heat in tissues, often caused by infection.

*Inflammatory bowel disease:* The broad term used to describe inflammation of the intestines for which the cause is unknown. The two major types of inflammatory bowel disease are Crohn's disease and ulcerative colitis.

*Inflammatory stricture:* A hardened scar caused by inflammation or infection.

*Internal anal sphincter:* An involuntary muscle in the anus which normally prevents the inadvertent loss of stool and gas.

*Internist:* A doctor who specializes in the diagnosis and non-surgical treatment of diseases.

*Intestines:* The organs in the digestive system which are located between the stomach and the anus and which help break down and absorb liquids and solid food. See also *Colon* and *Small intestine.*

*Keyhole deformity:* A crevice deformity of the anus in which the anus has the appearance of a keyhole and acts like a gutter through which liquids seep out.

*Laboratory method of biofeedback training:* In biofeedback training to treat fecal incontinence, this method uses the same balloon device used in colon motility studies.

*Large bowel.* See *Colon.*

*Large intestine.* See *Colon.*

*Machine-assisted biofeedback.* See *Electromyographic biofeedback.*

*Manometric tests.* See *Colon motility studies.*

*Manometry.* See *Colon motility studies.*

*Megacolon:* An enlarged colon associated with a large mass of retained stool which further stretches the colon.

*Megarectum.* An enlarged rectum associated with a large mass of retained stool which stretches the lining of the rectum.

*Mucus:* A thick, slippery secretion from the mucous membranes (such as the intestinal lining).

*Myelomeningocele* (also *meningomyelocele*): A severe form of spina bifida. See also *Spina bifida.*

*Nervous systems:* The voluntary nervous system and the involuntary nervous system are composed of the brain, the spinal cord, and sensory nerves, which provide messages to the brain from the body, and motor nerves, which provide messages from the brain to the muscles and which help the muscles function.

*Overflow incontinence* (also called *paradoxical diarrhea*): Soft or liquid stool that flows past a fecal impaction in the colon and rectum.

*Paradoxical diarrhea.* See *Overflow incontinence.*

*Pelvic floor muscles:* Muscles in the pelvic floor that normally assist in maintaining continence.

*Perineometer:* An instrument that displays the signals that are picked up by electrodes, the perineometer is used in electromyographic tests and in electromyographic biofeedback training.

*Peristalsis:* A series of involuntary muscle contractions in the esophagus and intestines which serve to move food along in the digestive system.

*Proctitis:* Inflammation of the rectum.

*Proctography.* See *Defecography.*

*Proctoscopy:* A diagnostic test for looking at the rectum through an instrument called a proctoscope.

*Proctosigmoidoscopy.* A diagnostic test for looking at the rectum and the sigmoid colon through an instrument called a sigmoidoscope.

*Pseudoincontinence:* Leakage of material other than stool from the rectum, or leakage of stool from an opening other than the rectum.

*Puborectalis muscle:* One of the muscles in the pelvic floor which forms a U-shaped loop around the rectum and normally assists in maintaining continence.

*Pudendal nerve neuropathy:* Injury to the pudendal nerve caused by stretching that impairs the function of that nerve.

*Rectal prolapse:* A condition in which the lining of the rectum becomes detached and slides down. An *internal prolapse* is not visible and may occur only during straining to have a bowel movement; an *external prolapse* protrudes from the rectum and may require surgical correction.

*Rectal saline infusion test:* A diagnostic test measuring the reservoir capacity of the rectum.

*Rectum:* An elastic segment of the bowel near its terminal end, consisting of smooth muscle. The rectum expands to accommodate stool and store it until defecation occurs.

*Sigmoid colon:* The S-shaped part of the large intestine.

*Sigmoidoscopy:* A diagnostic test for looking at the sigmoid colon through an instrument called a sigmoidoscope.

*Small intestine:* The organ in the digestive system connecting the stomach and the colon.

*Sonography.* See *Anorectal ultrasound*.

*Spina bifida:* A congenital defect in which the spinal cord does not close over properly. The most severe form is known as *myelomeningocele* or *meningomyelocele*.

*Stool.* See *Feces*.

*Stress incontinence:* The accidental and involuntary loss of urine, feces, or gas when coughing, sneezing, lifting, or doing anything else that puts pressure on the abdomen.

*Tenesmus:* An urgent sensation of needing to move the bowels, even when little stool is present and when little can be expelled.

*Tumor:* An abnormal overgrowth of tissue which may put pressure on the organs that are next to it.

*Ulcerative colitis.* See *Colitis.*

*Urge incontinence:* The accidental and involuntary loss of urine, feces, or gas when the person is aware of the need to get to the bathroom but is not able to hold the material long enough to get there.

*Urinary incontinence:* The accidental and involuntary loss of urine from the urinary sphincter.

*Valsalva maneuver:* The action of closing the airways and straining down on the abdominal muscles (such as when straining to have a bowel movement).

# Additional Resources

*For more information about incontinence:*

HIP (Help for Incontinent People)
P.O. Box 544, Union, SC 29379
803-579-7900

IFBD (International Foundation for Bowel Dysfunction)
P.O. Box 17864, Milwaukee, WI 53217
414-964-1799

The Simon Foundation for Continence
P.O. Box 815, Wilmette, IL 60091
708-864-3913

*For information about sexual health:*

Coalition on Sexuality and Disability
122 E. 23rd Street, New York, NY 10010
212-242-3900

Sex Information and Education Council of the U.S.
130 West 42nd Street, Suite 2500
New York, NY 10036
212-819-9770

*For more information about ostomy surgery and ostomy care:*
United Ostomy Association
36 Executive Park, Suite 120, Irvine, CA 92714
714-660-8624

# References

"Faecal Incontinence." Symposium moderated by F. M. Penninckx. *International Journal of Colorectal Disease* 2 (1987): 173-86.

James H. MacLeod. "Fecal Incontinence: A Practical Program of Management." *Endoscopy Review* (December 1988).

Marvin M. Schuster. "Fecal Incontinence." In *Medicine for the Practicing Physician,* 2d ed. Edited by J. W. Hurst. Stoneham, Mass., 1988.

———. "Biofeedback Control of Gastrointestinal Motility." In *Biofeedback: Principles and Practice for Clinicians,* 2d ed. Edited by J. V. Basmajian. Baltimore, 1983.

———, ed. *Proceedings of the Conference on Rehabilitation.* American Cancer Society, Maryland Division, 1979.

———. "Motor Action of Rectum and Anal Sphincters in Continence and Defecation." *Handbook of Physiology.* Edited by C. Code and C. Ladd Prosser. Baltimore, 1968.

J. F. Van Nostrand et al. *The National Nursing Home Survey: 1977 Summary for the United States.* Department of Health, Education, and Welfare Publication no. PHS 79-1794. Washington, D.C., 1979.

William E. Whitehead and Marvin M. Schuster. *Gastrointestinal Disorders: Behavioral and Physiological Basis for Treatment.* San Diego, 1985.

# Index

Page references appearing in *italic* type refer to illustrations.

Library of Congress Cataloging-in-Publication Data

Schuster, Marvin M. (Marvin Meier), 1929–
    Keeping control : understanding and overcoming fecal
incontinence
/ Marvin M. Schuster and Jacqueline Wehmueller.
        p.    cm.
Includes bibliographical references and index.
ISBN 0-8018-4915-2. — ISBN 0-8018-4916-0 (pbk.)
1. fecal incontinence—Popular works.    I. Wehmueller,
Jacqueline.
II. Title.
    RC866.D43S37    1994
616.3´42—dc20        94-8431    CIP